# Infection and Environment

# Infection and Environment

**Colin Kaplan**
*MSc, MB, ChB, Dip Bact, FIBiol, FRCPath*
*Emeritus Professor of Microbiology in the University of Reading*

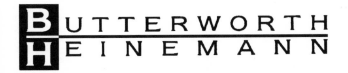

Butterworth-Heinemann
Linacre House, Jordan Hill, Oxford OX2 8DP
A division of Reed Educational and Professional Publishing Ltd

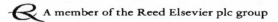 A member of the Reed Elsevier plc group

OXFORD   BOSTON   JOHANNESBURG
MELBOURNE   NEW DELHI   SINGAPORE

First published 1997

**British Library Cataloguing in Publication Data**
A catalogue record for this book is available from the British Library

**Library of Congress Cataloguing in Publication Data**
A catalogue record for this book is available from the Library of Congress

ISBN 0 7506 2740 9

Typeset by Bath Typesetting, Bath
Printed and bound in Great Britain by Biddles Ltd, Guildford and King's Lynn

# Contents

*This book is dedicated gratefully to the memory of
Harry Zwarenstein, Frank Forman and Marinus van den Ende
who, in their different ways, have exerted a deep and
continuing influence on me since my time as a student
and young Assistant Pathologist
in the University of Cape Town Medical School.*

# Preface

The sound practice of medicine is not always straightforward. Medicine, whether in general or specialist practice, of course requires clinical skills – history taking, physical examination, and so on; and also the knowledge to interpret the findings of these and any special investigations thought necessary. But more is needed. Practitioners ought to be aware of the flux of both infectious and non-infectious diseases in the communities they serve, and how these diseases are related to the social and physical environments of their patients. Doctors are, after all, involved in the ecology of their communities. They need, therefore, to be conscious of epidemiology; and an epidemiological approach should be helpful in their everyday affairs.

The significance of epidemiology to medical administrators and practitioners of public-health medicine is obvious, but the statistics which they consider are, in clinical medicine, transformed into individuals asking for help. That help will often be more swiftly available and more to the point when the doctor's diagnostic skills are fine-tuned by epidemiological awareness.

This book has its origin in my long-time interest in the ecology of communicable disease agents. As I note in the text, ecology is the study of the relationships and interactions of biological agents of all kinds with each other and the environments in which they find themselves. This, I believe, is different in kind from the operations known to some public-health epidemiologists as 'ecologic analysis' (see papers in the *American Journal of Public Health* 1994, **84**, 819–842). It is also a more correct use of the concept of ecology. Their use is connected with the collection and analysis of biological data of public-health interest. Data related to a community concerning a problem may give, when analysed, different results from data on the same subject related to individuals. This gives rise to what – in these circles – is known as 'the ecological fallacy', which is an arbitrary use of words worthy of Humpty Dumpty, and to the uninitiated is liable to give a wrong impression of the relationship between ecology and epidemiology.

The environments in which humans find themselves are complex, encompassing not only intrafamilial and interpersonal relationships, but also the social, economic, and moral climates in which they operate, as well as the physical environment – geographical, geomorphological, meteorological – and the biological including interactions with plants, pets, and other animals including (often very significantly) insects and other arthropods. Perturbations of some or all of these environmental components may be expected to impinge on some or all of the others, with consequential alterations in some or all of the interrelationships.

The concept of radiative forcing of climate change, i.e., global warming, made me look at some of the possible effects it may have on some infectious diseases. However the book is not devoted solely to this environmental aspect of infectious diseases. Nor is it intended as a compendium of all, or even many, of the changes which may occur as a result of global warming or alteration in any other environmental components. It is a personal view of some of the conditions which I believe are important now, and some of those which may become increasingly so.

The phenomenon of global warming has been officially recognized by governments. Reminders of some possible outcomes of the new circumstances may well be useful in keeping the guardians of the public health aware that the people – whose health it is – know that they may be at hazard; and knowing it, expect to see signs of protective activity. They will not for long accept mere soothing words from politicians.

I owe thanks to several people: my wife for her forbearance while I wrote the book; my son Lewis for his trenchant criticism of the style of the opening chapter – which I hope I have applied to the rest of the book; Dr R. Killick-Kendrick for help in understanding leishmanial ecology; and, by no means least, Professor Brian Hoskins for his invaluable help in advising me about the intricacies of forecasting the effects on climate of global warming – but the way that advice was used is not his responsibility, but mine.

Colin Kaplan
Reading, September 1996

# Chapter 1

# Epidemiology and ecology

Infectious diseases are caused by many different kinds of agents – bacteria, viruses, mycoplasmas, fungi, protozoa, worms. Their activities may be modified by diverse environmental factors – climate, poverty, overcrowding, intercurrent disease, malnutrition, as well as personal factors such as age, sex, immune status and so on. These are all ecological factors. Disease may be defined as any condition of imperfect functioning of the body resulting in observable signs and symptoms, and is an inevitable companion of life. Because living systems do not always work perfectly, and may also be attacked from without, disease is also an obligatory component of any ecosystem. The prospect of a disease-free world is therefore illusory, and the study of the causes of diseases and, more immediately, of infectious diseases, is necessary so that those diseases able to be cured can be successfully treated, and the effects of others can be ameliorated or prevented.

Because either the agent or the subject will win the contest, an infectious disease is an asymmetrical partnership between the infecting agent and the infected subject, and its occurrence is related to the environments in which the partners exist. An understanding of their ecology is not only helpful, but necessary, if effective means are to be deployed to control and prevent such diseases.

Ecology, as practised by professional ecologists, is the study of living organisms in their environments. The name is derived from the Greek *oikos*, a home or dwelling place. There are many components in an environment – geomorphological, climatic, biological – and organisms in an environment react with it by altering it physically or chemically, and by interacting with other organisms of all kinds in a shared habitat. Students of ecology therefore deal with interactive networks of great complexity – including both animate and inanimate components – which can be disturbed by many agencies acting either independently or together. A disturbed network of relationships means an altered ecology. Depending upon the type of alteration effected, this may result in a change in the epidemiology of an infectious disease. Epidemiology is thus, properly, a subdivision, but an important one, of ecology. Immunization, for example, which changes the potential habitat of a pathogen adversely in a highly specific way, will result in a reduction in the incidence and severity of disease caused by that pathogen: a change in the ecological relationship between host and parasite has altered the epidemiology of the disease.

Unlooked-for sequels are unlikely to occur if major activities are undertaken only when the ecology of a target area is well understood (Davis, 1963). A small, well-defined plague focus in the Little Karroo of the eastern Cape Province in South Africa was a candidate for eradication because of its proximity to Port Elizabeth, a rather densely populated industrial city. The rodent carrying plague in this focus was the gerbil *Desmodillus auricularis*. In a much larger neighbouring focus the carrier was *Otomys irroratus*. Since *Desmodillus* is found in open areas of firm ground and *Otomys* in bushy country, and *Otomys* is, in any case, too large to be able to enter and inhabit deserted gerbil burrows, it is very unlikely to colonize the gerbils' habitat. The risk of the plague focus being taken over and enlarged by the incursion of this other carrier was therefore considered to be negligible and the eradication of the *Desmodillus* focus to be safe (Dr E. K. Hartwig, personal communication). There are, however, examples of ignorant or unconsidered alterations of habitats causing grave problems to the public health, and also sometimes to wildlife, whether terrestrial or aquatic.

Alterations in macro-ecology may bring about changes in the distribution of pathogens and thus of the diseases they cause. The natural history of Lyme disease illustrates this very well (see below, and Chapter 9). There is – not always recognized frequently enough – the possibility that man-made changes in the ecology of a given area may do harm as well as the good aimed at. For example, the building of the Aswan High Dam in Egypt made more Nile water available for the irrigation of a greatly increased area, and hence an increase in food production. It also enlarged the habitat of the snail hosts of the schistosome worms which cause bilharzia; and, in addition, because nutrients carried by the river were prevented from reaching the sea, the fish stocks in the eastern Mediterranean were sadly impoverished.

The word *epidemiology* is derived from three words in classical Greek meaning 'knowledge of what is upon the people'. It has been defined in many ways, but perhaps the least cluttered and most useful is that given by MacMahon and Pugh (1970) – 'epidemiology is the study of the distribution and determinants of disease frequency in man'. Nowadays 'epidemiology' is frequently used instead of 'epizootiology' in relation to the diseases of animals. Sylvatic plague in rodents (see Chapter 9) offers a straightforward view of the relationship of ecology to epidemiology, however, the connection is not always so clear cut.

The study of the distribution of disease can be regarded as a counting exercise in which the numbers of people suffering from various diseases are totalled. The number with a specific disease at a particular time or brief interval of time indicates its *prevalence*, or how many cases have occurred. A more useful statistic is the *incidence rate* – the number of new cases which have occurred per some standard measure of population; e.g. $x\%$ or, more usually, $y$ per 100 000. To reach this sort of formulation we need to know not only the number of new cases during some specified period (the *numerator*), but also the size of the population at risk (the *denominator*). In countries with a well-developed statistical service denominators can be obtained from the latest census figures – or extrapolations from them, given a knowledge of birth and death rates. More information can be extracted from prevalence figures and incidence rates if they are analysed as stratified samples, i.e. in populations categorized in distinct segments by age, sex, socioeconomic status and so on. For example, differences in the prevalence of a disease or infection in different age groups can be used to decide when, and in which population groups, preventive measures – such as vaccination programmes – should be initiated.

Modern epidemiological methods are extraordinarily powerful in exposing the determinants of disease frequency, not only in infectious, but also non-infectious diseases. An outstanding example is the elucidation, beyond a doubt, of the central rôle of tobacco smoke in the pathogenesis of coronary heart disease and cancer of the lung. Epidemiology also supplies information essential for forecasting health-care requirements and for assessing the effects of policy decisions on the public health.

Infection and parasitism are inherent in the existence of heterotrophic life forms, but are not necessarily synonymous with disease. This has been known for many years, and was clearly shown in 1923 by Dudley when he investigated outbreaks of diphtheria among naval cadets at the Royal Naval College, Greenwich. He found that many of the cadets without signs of disease were carrying *Corynebacterium diphtheriae* in their throats, that is they were infected subclinically. They were, however, being naturally immunized against diphtheria by small amounts of diphtheria toxin secreted by the organisms; but bacteria transferred from the throats of such carriers were able to infect and cause disease in other cadets with no immunity.

In the 1950s, before the deployment of poliomyelitis vaccines, Melnick and his collaborators (Melnick and Ledinko, 1953; Melnick et al., 1955) established, by stratified serological surveys for poliomyelitis antibodies correlated with incidence rates of paralytic disease, that the ratio of subclinical infection to paralytic disease during epidemic outbreaks of poliomyelitis might range between 100:1 and 1000:1. Sero-epidemiology – especially by stratified surveys – remains a valuable technique in the investigation of infectious diseases.

A useful statistic which can be calculated from the study of death certificates is the *case fatality rate* of a particular disease (usually quoted as a percentage). Comparing the incidence and case fatality rates for a given disease over a defined period can tell us if its incidence and severity have changed. This is information which indicates the effectiveness of public-health measures such as vaccination programmes for the control of infectious diseases, and educational and other approaches to the control of conditions for which there is no vaccine, such as AIDS, or non-infectious conditions like coronary heart disease.

Epidemic outbreaks of virtually all infectious disease used to be easy to recognize because they tended to be large. However, today in developed countries, effective widespread vaccination against common infectious diseases has disqualified this approach for some of the diseases which may occur. Where, before vaccination, cases of disease would have been counted in hundreds, there may now be no more than a handful, as happens in polio and diphtheria outbreaks in well-vaccinated communities. When the usual expectation is of very few or no cases of, for example, polio in a year, five or six might be construed as an epidemic outbreak. This suggests that the key to the diagnosis of epidemic outbreaks is the recognition of an excess prevalence of the diseases in question. In the case of influenza, excess mortality from respiratory diseases in general is the main indicator that something is afoot. If the disease presents in an atypical clinical form, isolations of possible causative agents from, and antibody studies in, patients are used to confirm the outbreak and determine the agent responsible. This key fits even those diseases which are *endemic*, or always present in a population. For example, in Madras before the eradication of smallpox, the disease was endemic: several hundred cases were admitted to the Infectious Diseases Hospital in most years. However, when the number of admissions showed a clear increase, the authorities knew that they had an epidemic outbreak of smallpox to deal with (Dr A. R. Rao, personal communication). It was perhaps easier to make such a decision in Tamil Nadu State than in other places, where smallpox showed a distinct seasonal incidence, outbreaks occurring in winter and early spring. In Tamil Nadu temperature and humidity do not vary widely at different times of the year, and increased incidence of the disease did not have to be weighed against a possible seasonal increase in endemic infection – yet another example of the impingement of environmental factors on epidemiological findings.

The statistics of disease incidence tell us about the distributions of diseases, but they do not tell us the reasons for the observed distributions. These reasons are derived from 'the study of the ... determinants of disease frequency ...'; which is to say that a deeper understanding of the how and why of patterns of disease requires a knowledge of the causes of disease. The determinants of infectious disease necessarily include not only the causal agents, whether microorganisms or larger parasites, but also their *modus operandi* – the pathogenesis of the diseases they cause – and the defensive responses of the infected individual. These are part of *aetiology*, the study of causation, which, though clearly related to epidemiology, is not synonymous with it. In a narrow sense, aetiology is often taken to refer only to the immediate causal agent or factor. For example, *Mycobacterium tuberculosis* is the causal agent of tuberculosis, but the aetiology of tuberculosis is more complex than this simple statement suggests. As in various other infectious diseases, the presence of the organism, though necessary, is not always sufficient to ensure that infection progresses to recognizable disease.

The pathogenesis of a particular infectious disease may, for example, be conditional on the portal of entry of the pathogen; but for any given portal the process is pretty consistent. Although both bubonic and pneumonic plague are caused by the same pathogen, *Yersinia pestis*, their epidemiology in human beings is different. The former is spread from a rodent reservoir by intermediary fleas which are infected while feeding on their rodent hosts, and subsequently transfer from dead rodents to humans whom they infect while attempting to take blood meals. Patients with bubonic plague develop septicaemia and a few survive long enough for the circulating bacteria to invade the lungs and establish plague pneumonia. Patients with pneumonia excrete *Y. pestis* as an aerosol when they cough. Bacteria inhaled from the aerosol cloud are able to infect the lungs of susceptible subjects directly. The spread of infection by this route, from person to person, is more rapid than the indirect route by flea bites. The incubation period, probably being dose dependent, is not greatly different in the two types of clinical disease, ranging between 1 and 7 days, but the clinical course is more rapid and the outcome graver in pneumonic plague. The case fatality rate of untreated pneumonic plague approaches 100%, while that of the bubonic variety is between 30% and 50%. In septicaemic plague bacteria multiply in the circulating blood, and in some patients the clinical course may be astonishingly rapid. A person, apparently well at bed time, may be dead by morning, with none of the typical appearances associated with either bubonic or pneumonic plague; but he has, nevertheless, been killed by an overwhelming infection with *Y. pestis*.

A study of the distribution of a disease may give clues to its causation. The investigations of Dr John Snow, a London physician living in Soho, showed clearly that cholera, rampant in London in the mid-nineteenth century, was a water-borne disease. Even though the responsible microbial agent was not isolated and identified until almost 30 years later, Snow showed clearly the relationship between outbreaks of cholera and the environmental hazard presented by faecal contamination of water. His work is discussed more fully in Chapter 7, together with a closer examination of the impingement of environmental and climatic factors on the epidemiology of cholera.

From time to time reports appear of 'new' diseases. Some, recognized for the first time, are new, but some are old diseases which have re-emerged or been recognized in a different part of the world, perhaps in a new guise. The infection now known as Lyme disease is an example. This condition appeared in 1975 as a cluster of cases diagnosed as 'juvenile rheumatoid arthritis' in and around the town of Lyme in Connecticut (Steere *et al.*, 1977). The epidemiological study of this condition showed clearly the importance of ecological understanding (and field techniques) in clarifying the problems associated with the investigation of new diseases. The emergence of Lyme disease depended on incremental changes in the environment, and hence the ecology of the area, during 20 years or more. Lyme disease was virtually unrecognized before 1975, but it offers important insights into the relationships between human interventions in the physical environment and the appearance (or disappearance) of particular infections.

Since the Second World War, rabies in Europe has been overwhelmingly associated with the red fox, *Vulpes vulpes* (Kaplan *et al.*, 1986). Possibly because of the disruptions caused by the Second World War, the disease reached epizootic proportions in the European fox population, with a steady movement of the infection westwards from Poland and the former USSR. West Germany was heavily involved, with increasing numbers of rabid foxes causing measurable economic loss to farmers whose cattle were infected and either died or had to be destroyed. The disease moved from north-west Germany to Denmark, where, despite extensive destruction of foxes, successful control of its spread was only temporary. The West German authorities also instituted extensive destruction of foxes in attempts to control the disease, again with only short-term success.

In Switzerland, also seriously concerned by the presence of rabid foxes, the behavioural ecology of the animals was studied. The fox is a territorial animal. When individual territory holders die or are slaughtered their vacant territories are rapidly occupied by immigrant foxes, and the population of susceptibles is thus maintained. Swiss scientists, convinced that destruction of foxes would never lead to the control of vulpine rabies, developed an attenuated strain of rabies virus that could safely and effectively be used as a vaccine. Having also developed a delivery system they showed in a relatively small field trial that an epidemic outbreak was rapidly brought to a halt by vaccinating foxes ahead of the advancing front of infection. The fact that the ecological studies of foxes established that the animals were seldom, if ever, found above an altitude of 2000 metres somewhat reduced the difficulties of distributing baits containing the vaccine in mountainous regions. The size of the areas in which the vaccine was applied was steadily increased until, in a comparatively short time, the only fox rabies in Switzerland was at the borders with countries which still harboured many infected foxes.

Other countries cautiously followed the Swiss lead, with the result that 20 years after the introduction of an ecological approach to disease control, there is a remarkable diminution in vulpine rabies in western Europe. With an extension of this control method eastwards, there is now a good prospect that, even if it is not eradicated, wildlife rabies can at least be very closely limited.

Although myxomatosis is a disease of rabbits and not humans it is mentioned here for two reasons. It shows how the spread of an infection may be influenced by weather conditions and it offers a good example of the way the evolution of a pathogen can be modified by the ecosystem in which it operates. The two distinguishable varieties of myxoma virus and the closely related fibroma virus are native to the Americas, where biting insects transmit them mechanically within species of rabbits of the genus *Sylvilagus*, causing a generally non-lethal and unrecognized infection.

When transmitted to the European rabbit *Oryctolagus cuniculi*, classical myxoma viruses cause a severe, acute, highly lethal

infection. After a 14-year history of useful experimental studies on
the feasibility of using myxoma virus to control rabbit populations
in Australia, and a degree of bureaucratic reluctance to embark on
its use, a small-scale field experiment was instituted in the Murray
River catchment area in 1950 to determine whether or not it would
be able to reduce and control the size of wild rabbit populations.
The early stages of the experiment were decidedly unfruitful, but
while the field workers were deciding to abandon it, there were
heavy falls of rain in eastern Australia which led to widespread
flooding in the extensive basin of the Murray and Darling rivers and
their tributaries. This allowed free breeding and great enhancement
of mosquito populations which unexpectedly spread the virus like
wildfire among the rabbits of the entire combined catchment area.
Had 1950 been a year of El Niño (see Chapter 7), the experimental
introduction of myxomatosis may well have failed. Occurrences of
El Niño are not only likely to lead to the failure of the south-east
monsoon in India, but also to droughts in south-eastern Africa and
eastern Australia – in which case the intense flush of mosquitoes, so
necessary for success, would not have happened.

In the early months of the epizootic spread, kill rates among
rabbit populations approached 100%. Although the intensity of the
outbreak came as a surprise to the Australian authorities, a long-
term study of the effects of the introduction was set up (Fenner and
Ratcliffe, 1965). Not only were the results produced of great interest
concerning the evolution of myxomatosis of rabbits, but also of
considerable consequence in the study of infectious diseases in
general.

The early and rapid success of myxomatosis in reducing rabbit
numbers in Australia, encouraged a private citizen in France, Dr A.
Delille, to introduce the virus into his 250-hectare walled estate at
Maillebois, in central France. The introduction was made in mid-
June 1952. By the end of August, not only was Delille's estate
practically free of rabbits, but there had been outbreaks of
myxomatosis as far as 45 kilometres from Maillebois. By the
summer of 1953 the disease had been recorded in most of western
Europe; it was confirmed in southern England (Kent) in October
1953 and rapidly spread to most of Britain.

As the years passed the kill rate in Australia became steadily
smaller. The study directed by Fenner (Fenner and Ratcliffe, 1965)
found that this resulted from a combination of reduced virulence of
the virus and increased resistance of the rabbits. In France and
Britain, too, kill rates were reduced, but the virulence of British
strains of the virus was less attenuated than that of French strains.
In both Australia and France epidemic outbreaks of myxomatosis

are seasonal. In addition, domestic hutch rabbits in France were extensively affected. This is not so in Britain, where not only have domestic rabbits been infected rarely, but seasonality is less marked, and outbreaks often seem to be restricted by fences and other mechanical barriers to the movements of rabbits, with populations of uninfected rabbits being found next to heavily infected areas.

The epidemiological differences between myxomatosis in Britain and in Australia and France suggested that different transmission mechanisms were operating. In Australia mosquitoes are the most important carriers and spreaders of the virus. There are no rabbit fleas. Mosquitoes are also important in France in the summer, with fleas of minor significance in the winter. In Britain, mosquitoes are less important in spreading the infection, with a much greater part being played by the rabbit flea *Spilopsyllus cuniculi*, an efficient vector.

The sustained higher kill rate in Britain may be partly explained by the fact that, unlike in Australia, there is less strong evidence of genetically resistant rabbits. This probably results from a combination of causes. Outbreaks of disease occur irregularly, both geographically and in time, and this tends to minimize the selection for resistance. In some parts of France, for example, where there had been no outbreaks for several years, rabbits, when tested, were fully susceptible to myxomatosis. In both France and Britain there is a higher proportion of more virulent strains of virus circulating than in Australia. After an outbreak of the disease there is thus a smaller proportion of immune survivors available for breeding.

The difference in Britain probably also has to do with the fact that a significant proportion of outbreaks occurs in winter when, as was shown experimentally in Australia (Marshall, 1959), a greater mortality occured at lower temperatures – 0–4°C in Marshall's experiments. The type of vector is also important. In winter, mosquitoes are not active, but fleas are, and they tend not to desert living hosts, but they do leave dead ones. Fleas therefore transmit virus of proven lethality. At the relatively low temperatures of British winters even moderately attenuated strains of virus would kill. Transmission by fleas, while not selecting absolutely for strains of high virulence, does, nevertheless, select against strains permitting survival of infected rabbits. Rabbits infected with attenuated strains of virus live longer, and where mosquitoes are the main vectors of infection, there is a high probability that insects feeding on sick rabbits will pick up and transmit viruses which either will not kill the next rabbit infected, or will do so after inducing a clinically milder and longer lasting disease.

This view is supported by the relatively high proportion of

virulent strains (Grades I and II) in Britain 8 or 9 years after the introduction of the virus. This is to be compared with the situation in Australia where, at comparable times, strains of Grade I virulence were not isolated, but Grades II and III were common, and 5 years later Grade II was barely represented while 60% of isolates were of Grade III virulence. Nevertheless, with the passage of time, changes similar to those previously noted in Australia and France began to be seen in Britain. During the 4-year period from 1966 to 1969, young wild rabbits were captured and held until their maturity. They were then infected with standard doses of a strain of myxoma virus which killed 90–95% of laboratory rabbits of a line not previously exposed to the virus. The mortality rates of the wild rabbits were not much different from those of the laboratory rabbits, but they survived longer until death. A similar investigation was made between 1970 and 1976. In 1970 the mortality in wild rabbits was 59%, in 1974, 17% and in 1976, 20%. These findings indicated an increase in the innate resistance of wild rabbits to the virus (Ross and Sanders, 1977). A field investigation in 1989 showed that strains of virus isolated from rabbits naturally infected during an outbreak of myxomatosis were almost all of virulence grade IIIA (in a range where grade I is most virulent with a mortality rate of c. 95%, and grade V is least virulent) (Ross *et al.*, 1989). Innate resistance of rabbits thus continues to increase and case fatality rates to decrease, indicating evolutionary changes in both host and pathogen.

In their natural *Sylvilagus* hosts the myxoma viruses infect but only very exceptionally cause disease, and may be regarded as having attained climax states. This is not yet so in *Oryctolagus*, although it may be expected to happen in the future. The necessary changes in the genetics of both rabbits and myxoma virus will, however, occur at very different rates in Australia and Britain (with France perhaps taking an intermediate position) because the ecosystems in which the disease operates differ in such a major factor as the transmission mechanism, and it is this which, in myxomatosis, appears to provide the selection pressure which drives the evolutionary process.

Zoonotic infections are by no means uncommon although, without doubt, more remain to be uncovered. The rational control of such infections – especially in the absence of effective vaccines – depends heavily on an understanding of the ecology of the infective agent and its reservoir host(s). Lassa fever in Nigeria, and other haemorrhagic fevers in South America, are caused by members of the arenavirus group and are known to have reservoirs in various rodents which, from time to time, come into contact with humans.

The basis for a rational programme to prevent human infection thus exists; however, the full-scale implementation of such a programme is unlikely because of the costs it would generate and the relatively undeveloped rural environment in which it would have to be implemented. The severe haemorrhagic diseases caused by infection with the filoviruses of Marburg and Ebola fevers point to a further difficulty in control. Both of these highly fatal infections of humans appear to have been spread from monkeys, but among the scientists who have investigated the diseases and their causative viruses, there is a strong feeling that monkeys are not the reservoir of infection, but secondary hosts. Effective control measures depend on a knowledge of the reservoir host(s) and transmission mechanisms of the agents; which is to say that more must be learned of their ecology, which will be both expensive and time consuming. However, until more is known of the ecology of these agents, the only effective measure available for control of the diseases they cause is the old-fashioned one of strict quarantine of all involved in outbreaks. Such a procedure may be reasonably successful in isolated villages in the African bush where previous outbreaks have occurred, but in the context of large conurbations (whether Third- or First-World) the efficacy of such a tactic must be doubted.

# References

Davis, D.H.S. (1963). Ecology and vector control. *Bulletin of the World Health Organization* **26**, Supplement, 127–133.

Dudley, S.F. (1923). *Special Report Series of the Medical Research Council* No. 75, London.

Fenner, F. and Ratcliffe, F.N. (1965). *Myxomatosis*. Cambridge University Press, London.

Kaplan, C., Turner, G.S., and Warrell D.A. (1986). *Rabies the Facts*. Oxford University Press, Oxford.

MacMahon, B.M. and Pugh, T.F. (1970). *Epidemiology: Principles and Methods*. Little, Brown & Co, Boston.

Marshall, I.D. (1959). The influence of ambient temperature on the course of myxomatosis in rabbits. *Journal of Hygiene*, Cambridge **57**, 484–497.

Melnick, J.L. and Ledinko, N. (1953). Development of neutralizing antibodies against the three types of poliomyelitis virus during an epidemic period: the ratio of inapparent infection to clinical poliomyelitis. *American Journal of Hygiene* **58**, 207–222.

Melnick, J.L., Paul, J.R. and Walton, M. (1955). Serologic epidemiology of poliomyelitis. *American Journal of Public Health* **45**, 429–437.

Ross, J. and Sanders, M.F. (1977). Innate resistance to myxomatosis in wild rabbits in England. *Journal of Hygiene*, Cambridge **79**, 411–415.

Ross, J., Tittensor, A.M., Fox, A.P. and Sanders, M.P. (1989). Myxomatosis in farmland rabbit populations in England and Wales. *Epidemiology and Infection* **103**, 333–357.

Steere, A.C., Malawista, S.E., Snydman, D. *et al.* (1977). Lyme arthritis: an epidemic of oligo-articular arthritis in children and adults in three Connecticut communities. *Arthrology and Rheumatism* **20**, 7–17.

# Chapter 2

# Pathogenesis of disease and defence against pathogens

Some knowledge of the pathogenesis of infectious diseases is necessary for a sound understanding of their epidemiology. Bubonic and pneumonic plague have different epidemiologies (see Chapter 1) because *Yersinia pestis*, having a different portal of entry for each of these clinical conditions, initiates the diseases by infecting different anatomical environments, which sets in train different pathogenetic sequences. This chapter is necessarily brief, and is certainly an incomplete sketch of pathogenetic processes. An extremely satisfactory account of the ways infectious diseases develop is given in *The Pathogenesis of Infectious Disease* (Mims, 1987).

To be able to cause disease and be, so to say, a professional pathogen a microorganism must not only be transmissible, but also invasive. There are a few apparent exceptions to this statement. *Clostridium botulinum*, for example, causes disease when a subject ingests the botulism toxin secreted in a contaminated foodstuff, and the bacteria need never enter the body of the victim; but virtually all the toxins which are important parts of the pathogenetic armamentarium of many microorganisms are produced *in situ* in the tissues of the infected host. Some organisms, such as *Yersinia pestis*, can only produce the full range of toxic products at the body temperature of an infected mammal.

A very extensive range of factors is available to most microbial pathogens, which promote their invasiveness and enable them to neutralize or overcome the protective mechanisms of the host. Although most pathogens operate in the tissues of the infected subject, in some – even very dangerous – infections the invasion may be extremely limited. In diphtheria, for example, the bacteria are confined to the tough pseudomembrane of fibrin and inflammatory cells which forms in the upper respiratory tract, or on superficial wounds of the skin. The toxin elaborated is absorbed from the production site and carried in the circulation to distant targets such as the heart and other organs where it becomes fixed to cells and damages them by inhibiting protein synthesis. Involvement of neurones may lead to late paralyses in patients with diphtheria.

The disease can be both treated and prevented by diphtheria antitoxin in the absence of any specific antibacterial therapy, which demonstrates that the toxin is indeed the major aggressive factor involved in the pathogenesis of diphtheria.

*Clostridium tetani* is another potentially lethal pathogen which acts at a distance. When the heat-resistant spores of *Cl. tetani* contaminate a wound they require a low redox potential (i.e. an anaerobic environment) to enable them to germinate, multiply as vegetative organisms, and secrete their toxin. Such environments are found in deep penetrating wounds, and wounds in which there is much necrotic tissue. The organism needs no further invasion than this to be able to kill its host. Other clostridia, such as those responsible for gas gangrene (of which *Cl. welchii*, although not the only one, is numerically the most important), produce necrotizing toxins in the tissues which will become gangrenous as a result. The primary defence against toxic infections such as diphtheria and tetanus is a sufficient concentration of circulating specific antitoxic antibody, acquired either naturally by previous infection (possibly subclinical), as may happen in diphtheria, or by artificial active immunization such as is possible with tetanus or diphtheria toxoids.

The first line of defence against infection with truly invasive microorganisms is phagocytosis by neutrophil polymorphonuclear leucocytes (neutrophils). This is an early manifestation of inflammation, which is pre-eminently a protective mechanism. When inflammation is inadequately controlled, however, it may become remarkably destructive of host tissues, especially when acting in concert with immune responses, as may occur in chronic infections such as tuberculosis and leprosy, and in some conditions such as rheumatoid arthritis in which infection – although suspected by some workers – has not been unequivocally demonstrated.

Many pathogens secrete exotoxins of one sort or another, some which disable defensive cells and enable the pathogen to invade the host's tissues. However, not all are directly destructive of these cells. *Vibrio cholerae*, for example – which does not enter the gut cells, but colonizes their surfaces – causes disease when its potent enterotoxin attaches itself to enteral cells and disrupts the management of $Na^+$ and $Cl^-$ by causing an overproduction of cyclic AMP, which leads to the loss from the blood of a large volume of isotonic fluid. If this is not corrected rather rapidly the patient is likely to die of hypovolaemic shock. In cholera and other conditions caused by enterotoxins of cholera type, for example travellers' diarrhoeas induced by toxinogenic strains of *Escherichia coli*, the protective actions of inflammation are inoperative because the microorganisms remain in the lumen of the gut, where they are not invasive, *sensu stricto*, and the inflammatory response is unable to reach them.

There are many different mechanisms of microbial pathogenicity. Several of the more important or more frequently observed are mentioned elsewhere in this book. Toxins are produced by many pathogens and play important rôles in the genesis of the diseases caused by the microbes which produce them. Many of the most potent are exotoxins which are secreted by the living organisms and enter the fluids and tissues of the infected host where they exert their pathogenic effects. Most, but not all, of the best-known exotoxins are products of Gram-positive organisms, especially of the genus *Clostridium*. A potent exotoxin, active in both the gut and the nervous system, is produced by the Gram-negative organism *Shigella dysenteriae*. Indeed, many Gram-negative enteropathogens secrete enterotoxins as the basis of their pathogenicity. Exotoxins interfere with vital activities of cells, as in diphtheria, killing them; or they inhibit essential neural functions, as in tetanus and botulism, leading to paralyses or other major malfunctions. Some toxins may intensify the effects of other pathogenicity factors; for example, pertussis toxin seems to augment the adherence of *Bordetella pertussis* to mammalian cells. Those exotoxins which have been adequately studied exhibit either enzymic activity of one sort or another, or they inhibit important enzymes of the host; or they may be inserted into host-cell membranes as pores, allowing abnormal entry and exit of solutes, leading to intracellular ionic imbalance, and disturbance, if not disruption, of function. The adherence of microbes to their target cells is an important pathogenetic mechanism. This may be achieved by the action of adhesins carried on the surface of the microorganism, or by its attachment to the cell surface by pili – filamentous structures carried by many bacteria, some of which are non-pathogenic. Once adherent, the bacteria are enabled to enter the target cell by the action of invasins.

Bacterial capsules, also important factors in the pathogenicity of bacteria, are mostly polysaccharides, as exemplified by the pneumococci and meningococci. These capsules are antiphagocytic; and, by virtue of structural differences and the different sugars of which they consist, confer serological specificity on the microorganisms. Immunity to one serotype of pneumococcus, for example, does not prevent infection by other types. Pneumococcal capsules also seem to be associated, not simply with pathogenicity, but also with virulence – the severity of the disease caused by the infection. Eighty-four different pneumococcal serotypes are recognized. Some – especially type 3 – are more virulent than others. Most pneumococci are still sensitive to penicillin, but the number of strains resistant to penicillin, cephalosporins, and other antibiotics is increasing. Even in patients infected with penicillin-sensitive strains, the mortality may vary from about 5% with serotype 1, to about 50% with serotype 3, despite early treatment with large doses of penicillin or other suitable antibiotic.

Not all bacterial capsules are polysaccharides. The capsule of *Bacillus anthracis* consists of polyglutamic acid, while that of *Yersinia pestis* – a Gram-negative organism – is also proteinaceous. The capsule of *Y. pestis* plays a complex part in determining both pathogenicity and the virulence of the organism. The capsule, consisting of a surface antigen called Fraction 1, inhibits phagocytosis in infected animals. It is a phenotypic component whose production is determined by the temperature of incubation. In blocked fleas, i.e. infected fleas in which the proventriculus is occluded by a dense growth of *Y. pestis*, the organisms – at the temperature of the flea – produce pathogenicity factors V and W, but not Fraction 1, the antiphagocytic capsular substance. When such a flea attempts to take a blood meal from a mammalian host, the blood it ingests, unable to enter the proventriculus, is regurgitated into the skin of the host, carrying with it an inoculum of bacteria. In the host, at 37°C, the bacteria multiply, producing not only V and W, but also Fraction 1 which, in concert with the other known factors, confers on them full pathogenicity.

Several mechanisms allow pathogenic bacteria to elude the immune response of the host. They may carry surface receptors which bind host proteins, thus disguising themselves, or they may undergo rapid antigenic variation, making the host's immune responses nugatory, or their capsules may ward off the action of antibodies by preventing access to the bacterial cell.

When infecting Gram-negative microbes die, their cell walls disintegrate, producing endotoxin which promotes several important reactions in the infected person, such as fever and shock – especially of the kind known as toxic shock. Toxins and some other bacterial products such as capsular substances are able to inhibit phagocytosis. Some bacteria, for example *Brucella* spp., are able to withstand the killing powers of phagocytes, even after being engulfed, and use the phagocytic cells (especially macrophages) as carriers to spread them to distant parts of the body.

An appreciable number of microorganisms, although not regularly pathogenic, can cause disease when they are enabled – often by the lack of protective or defensive factors in the host – to invade individuals normally completely resistant to them. These organisms, described as opportunistic pathogens, for obvious reasons, tend to establish themselves in new environmental niches which emerge as a result of changing social conditions or the development of new technologies. *Legionella pneumophila* and several organisms of the same genus are able to invade pulmonary tissue and cause the pneumonia of legionnaires' disease (Fraser *et al.*, 1977). There is another clinical condition caused by *L. pneumophila* – Pontiac fever – in which the salient features are high fever, headache and myalgia (Glick *et al.*, 1978). Unlike the pneumonic form which carries a fatality rate of up to 20% in the absence of appropriate treatment, Pontiac fever appears to be non-lethal and probably involves fewer body systems than does legionnaires' disease. It was first recognized in 1968 when 144 persons developed symptoms after entering a government building (the Pontiac Building) while the air conditioning was working, although none became ill when it was not. Transmission was clearly airborne. The outbreak began about 3 weeks after groundworks close to the building had raised clouds of dust which enveloped the building, presumably contaminating the cooling water of the air-conditioning plant. The causative organism was isolated several years later from the lung tissue of guinea-pigs which had developed pneumonia after exposure in the building (Kaufmann *et al.*, 1981). Because these two rather different clinical types are caused by the same bacterium, infection with it is generally referred to as legionellosis. The factors which confer pathogenicity on *Legionella* may include a toxic protein, an endotoxin, and the ability to multiply in, and kill, macrophages which have phagocytosed them. Smoking, excess consumption of alcohol, and immune deficit all reduce resistance to the bacteria and increase the chances of infection and the development of legionellosis.

*Legionella* organisms have been isolated from mud and soil, but are mainly associated with water, especially in the taps supplying baths and showers (Fraser-Hoch *et al.*, 1981), and the water in the cooling towers of air-conditioning systems (Dondero *et al.*, 1980). Such contaminated sources are likely to give rise to common-source outbreaks, such as have been associated with hospitals, hotels, and air-conditioned buildings, where air-borne spread of the microbes appears to be the usual route of infection, although sporadic cases have been documented.

Legionellosis, in the form of legionnaires' disease, made a dramatic entry in 1976. At a convention of the American Legion at a hotel in Philadelphia, 221 of those attending developed various febrile pulmonary diseases, but the major clinical picture was that of pneumonia (Fraser *et al.*, 1977). There were 34 deaths. Since then, many common-source outbreaks of pneumonic legionellosis have been described, as well as many sporadic outbreaks. There is no compelling evidence that person-to-person transmission occurs, but some of those in contact with patients, such as medical and nursing attendants, may occasionally develop antibodies to the organisms. With the isolation of the organism and the development of reasonably reliable diagnostic tests, retrospective diagnoses of legionella infections have been made dating back to 1943 (Tatlock, 1944). There is no reason to doubt that such infections occurred even earlier. The documented epidemic outbreaks may have arisen because of changes in the ecology both of the organism and of humans, caused by technological change. A significant feature of outbreaks, as opposed to sporadic cases, is that they are common-source phenomena dependent on the presence of air conditioning in buildings, or relatively large numbers of water taps and shower roses capable of generating aerosol clouds of water droplets small enough to penetrate deep into the lung when inspired by a potential victim. Common-source outbreaks do not seem to have occurred before air conditioning of buildings became common. Prevention of such outbreaks clearly depends on the proper maintenance of air-conditioning systems, and especially cooling towers, to ensure that *Legionella* organisms do not multiply to such concentrations that they become a public-health hazard.

A pathogen entering a tissue makes a primary lodgement and does some damage. When cells are damaged by any of a wide variety of agents such as mechanical injury, ionizing or ultraviolet irradiation, heat or severe cold, or chemicals such as acids and alkalis, and, of course, invading microorganisms, the body reacts by mounting an inflammatory response. Inflammation is primarily protective, but when, for various possible reasons, it is extremely severe or continues for a long time, it may become destructive and cause disease even more serious than that which it was started to control. Rheumatoid arthritis is a prime example of the destructive aspect of inflammation.

Most inflammation is *acute*, i.e. of short duration, though it may be relatively mild or very severe. When a microbe invades the body it damages or kills some of the cells of the tissue in which it lodges. The cells release several pharmacologically active substances, including various prostaglandins, which set in train the inflammatory process. Among the first things to happen is dilatation of the local capillary blood vessels. More blood enters the damaged region, which therefore looks redder and feels warmer than normal. The walls of the capillaries become more porous than normal and blood plasma passes freely into the tissue spaces between cells, causing the part to swell. As the swelling increases, the injured or invaded part becomes painful. The damaged cells and the invading microorganisms both produce chemotactic substances which attract the phagocytic neutrophil polymorphs.

The neutrophils initially line the capillary walls and then work their way through the joins between the endothelial cells which constitute the vessel wall. When they enter the tissue spaces the cells move towards the bacteria and engulf them. Many different kinds of bacteria are killed and digested by this phagocytosis. In the best possible outcome, the invasion is halted and the episode is resolved. Some bacteria, however, are armed with substances which either make them very difficult to ingest or which, either before or after they are ingested, kill the neutrophils. Many of these substances are toxins; several, for example the toxins of *Bacillus anthracis* and *Bordetella pertussis*, are able to increase the concentration of cyclic AMP in host cells and disrupt the control of fluid and electrolyte concentrations. The *B. pertussis* toxin, which is active in neutrophils, is able to reduce their antibacterial activity and allow the invasion of the microbes to continue unimpeded. Many toxins are enzymes able to attack and damage important cell structures and components.

The earliest stages of inflammation and natural active immunization are closely related, both in time and in some of the cells involved. Previous infection by the same sort of bacteria should normally have caused an immune response. A second or subsequent infection acts as a further stimulus and the immune system makes a secondary or anamnestic response with the production of large amounts of specific antibodies which deal with the offensive armamentarium of the bacteria by neutralizing substances which destroy neutrophils, or by coating the bacteria with opsonic antibodies to make them more palatable to the neutrophils, or by destroying any protective coating they may have. The neutrophils, both living and killed, together with bacteria (alive or dead), and fluid exuded from the blood vessels, make up the pus which is so significant a part of many acute inflammations.

When the bacterial invasion is brought rapidly under control and the tissue or part is completely restored to its original state, the inflammation ends by *resolution*. When it is not quelled rapidly there is often some destruction of the host's tissues. Depending on the type of bacterial invader and the length of time that the inflammation persists, the damage may be either minor or quite extensive. Under these circumstances when the bacterial invasion (or other damaging event) is eventually overcome the damage is repaired – but not necessarily 'made good' – by a process which fills large gaps with fibrous, or scar, tissue. Inflammation ending by *repair*, may – depending on how much destruction there was – leave the tissue or part with a reduced function because of the amount of scar tissue present, or with virtually unimpaired function.

There are two other possible outcomes of acute inflammation. One is death. If the damage, however caused, is so rapid and severe that a vital function is compromised beyond correction then the subject will die. Several bacterial infections are able to do this – meningococcal and plague septicaemias are pre-eminent examples; but the acute inflammation of pneumococcal pneumonia may involve so much of the lungs that adequate gas exchanges are not possible and the patient dies from anoxia. The other is development into *chronic inflammation*.

Chronic inflammation is inflammation of long duration. It is characterized by the presence of large concentrations of mono-nuclear cells – lymphocytes and macrophages. There are two types of chronic inflammation. One is acute inflammation which has persisted for several weeks. Staphylococci are particularly prone to initiate pyogenic infections with the typical cellular infiltrations of acute inflammation. When infection is not eradicated promptly, which is a highly probable event in staphylococcal osteitis, for example, the neutrophils are joined by mononuclear cells – macrophages and lymphocytes. In peptic ulcers the lesions show a mixture of acute and chronic inflammation with mononuclear cells in the base of the ulcer and neutrophils infiltrating the edges.

The functions of the mononuclear cells are related but different. Macrophages are phagocytic cells which enter the inflammatory field relatively late. They ingest and sometimes destroy invading microparasites and other foreign material, but have a crucial immune function as well. They process the antigens of invading microbes and present them to the appropriate CD4 T lymphocytes, which then either promote the production of killer or cytotoxic T cells, or stimulate the matching B cells to produce antibodies specific to the invaders. Antibody-secreting B lymphocytes appear as plasma cells in histological sections of inflamed tissues. The antibodies involved in protection are the immune globulins referred to as IgM, IgG and IgA.

The other type of chronicity – granulomatous inflammation – is seen in the characteristic lesion of tuberculosis – the tubercle. The granuloma consists of a dense collection of cells of several provenances: neutrophils, eosinophils, macrophages, lymphocytes, plasma cells and fibroblasts, all – in their appropriate ways – going about their business of phagocytosis, or immune response, or forming scar tissue. Especially in tuberculotic granulomas, macro-phages differentiate into giant cells and epithelioid cells which are found in the centre of the tubercle surrounded by lymphocytes and fibroblasts. In tuberculosis the fate of the tubercle depends largely on the degree of immunity of the host. The pathogenesis of tuberculosis, and its relationship with the dissemination of tuberculous infection, is discussed in Chapter 4.

The immunity generated in response to infection depends largely on the pathogenetic habit of the infecting organism. *Corynebacterium diphtheriae*, *Vibrio cholerae*, *Clostridium tetani*, and other microbes which operate through the activity of their exotoxins, stimulate a predominantly humoral response. Because both diphtheria and tetanus toxins are blood borne, antitoxic antibody, in sufficient concentration, is highly efficient in preventing their deleterious effects. Cholera toxin, however, enters directly into the enteral cells susceptible to its action and is, therefore, effectively shielded from the action of antitoxic antibody. Survivors of mucosal infections with, for example, *V. cholerae*, produce IgA which is transported through mucosal cells and is active on their surfaces. The resulting immunity lasts for perhaps 3 years, during which time the secretory IgA will be able to prevent all but overwhelmingly large infections from colonizing the small-gut brush border. Viruses which infect their hosts via the blood stream – those spread by blood-feeding insects, for example, or those in which an early viraemia occurs after infection – can be dealt with by adequate concentrations of neutralizing antibody in the blood. When cells of target organs have been infected, however, cellular immune mechanisms are brought into play.

Immunization, by adversely altering the potential environment of a pathogen, can protect an individual against the development of disease; but individual immunity does not, of itself, offer protection against epidemic outbreaks of disease to a community or population. Such protection depends on the existence of *herd immunity*, which is determined by the immunity of a large enough proportion of the population preventing the free transmission in it of the infectious agent. This proportion, though high, is not necessarily the same for all pathogens, nor – for any single pathogen – the same for a wide range of population densities (Arita *et al.*, 1986). In the later stages of the smallpox eradication programme in India, when the disease was all but abolished in most of the country, there were persistent outbreaks in both Uttar Pradesh and Bihar States. These outbreaks threatened to vitiate the success so far achieved by the programme of surveillance and containment by immunization, which had been effective in much of the rest of India and the rest of the world. Administrative weaknesses in the health services of these States had led to a situation where smallpox virus was circulating in a large, unrecognized group of unvaccinated individuals – widows, the indigent and many Untouchables – despite figures which suggested that the overall acceptance rate for vaccination was satisfactorily high. When the true state of affairs was realized, heroic efforts were made to find and isolate cases of smallpox and vaccinate contacts. The system of surveillance and containment, vigorously applied to the whole population in these Indian States, successfully increased herd immunity to a level which effectively broke the chain of transmission of the virus.

Immunity in the control of epidemic infection is dealt with in specific detail in later chapters devoted to particular diseases or types of infection.

# References

Arita, I., Wickett, J. and Fenner, F. (1986). Impact of population on immunization programmes. *Journal of Hygiene*, Cambridge **96**, 459–466.

Dondero Jr, T. J., Rendtdorff, R.C., Mallinson, G.F. *et al.* (1980). Outbreak of Legionnaires' disease associated with a contaminated air conditioning cooling tower. *New England Journal of Medicine* **302**, 425–431.

Fraser, D.W., Tsai, T.F., Orenstein, W. *et al.* (1977). Legionnaires' disease: description of an epidemic of pneumonia. *New England Journal of Medicine* **297**, 1189–1197.

Fraser-Hoch, S.P., Bartlett, C.L.R., Tobin, J. O'H *et al.* (1981). Investigation and control of an outbreak of Legionnaires' disease in a district general hospital. *Lancet* **i**, 932–936.

Glick, T.H., Gregg, M.B., Berman, B. *et al.* (1978). Pontiac fever: an epidemic of unknown etiology In a health department. I. Clinical and epidemiologic aspects. *American Journal of Epidemiology* **107**, 149–160.

Kaufmann, A.F., McDade. J.E., Patton, C.M. *et al.* (1981). Pontiac fever: isolation of the etiologic agent (*Legionella pneumophila*) and demonstration of its mode of transmission. *American Journal of Epidemiology* **114**, 337–347.

Mims, C.A. (1987). *The Pathogenesis of Infectious Disease*, 3rd ed. Academic Press, London.

Tatlock, H. (1944). A rickettsia-like organism recovered from guinea pigs. *Proceedings of the Society for Experimental Biology and Medicine* **57**, 95–99.

# Chapter 3

# Measles, mumps and rubella

Measles and mumps are caused by infection with very specialized paramyxoviruses. The virus which causes rubella, despite being classified as a toga virus because it is an enveloped RNA virus, has no known relationship with other togaviruses such as yellow fever and dengue viruses, and the large number of other insect-borne, enveloped RNA viruses. The three diseases are dealt with in this chapter for the simple reason that modern practice aims to immunize against them with a combined measles, mumps, and rubella vaccine (MMR).

## Measles

Measles virus is related serologically to the viruses of the animal diseases rinderpest and distemper. It has a genome consisting of a single molecule of single-stranded RNA. Geographically widely separated viruses show no important strain variations. Why this should be is unclear: the influenza B myxovirus, also with a genome consisting of a single molecule of RNA, undergoes slow antigenic drift. That measles virus does not, has the great advantage that a universally used vaccine strain may be expected to confer immunity against all current epidemic strains of the virus.

In unvaccinated or inadequately vaccinated populations measles is primarily a disease of childhood except in small, isolated societies which are in contact with members of large populations only intermittently and at fairly long intervals. Under such conditions, measles attacks all age groups. This was documented very clearly by the work of Peter Panum, a Danish physician who helped to care for the population of the Faroë Islands during an outbreak of measles in 1846. He made two very important observations. The first was that, between the exposure of a subject to a patient in the early stages of measles and the appearance of his rash, there was a period of about 14 days. This was so uniform that Panum believed that the disease developed only as a result of contact with patients with the disease. The second was that the outbreak, although very widespread in the population, did not include people 67 years old or older. When he enquired, Panum learned that there had been a previous outbreak of measles in the islands in 1780 when, just as in the present outbreak, almost everybody had been affected. This observation indicates (to us) that immunity to measles is very durable, and probably life-long. It also indicates that the causal agent – measles virus – is unable to establish itself in a small, isolated population. This has been confirmed in other island and isolated communities, such as the population of Greenland, Inuit communities in the far north of Canada, and isolated Amerind tribes in the Amazon basin. The smallest population able to sustain endemic measles is about 500 000 (Black, 1965). In smaller populations introduced virus causes widespread epidemic disease in all age groups, except those immunized by a previous outbreak, and then disappears.

The infection is spread by the aerial route when the infected subject generates aerosol clouds of virus by coughing and sneezing. In unvaccinated communities the infection rate in any epidemic outbreak is generally very high, approaching 98% of those lacking immunity. In developed countries such as those of western Europe and North America mortality from measles is very small – considerably less than 1%. In Third World countries, however, deaths of children from measles are numerous. In parts of Africa and South America, for example, case fatality rates of 30% or more have been recorded. Some attribute this to genetic differences between Third World and First World children. There is some evidence for this relating to Amerinds of the Amazon basin (Neel *et al.*, 1970; Black *et al.*, 1971), but elsewhere it is more likely to be due to differences in nutrition and general hygiene, which may well include the incidence of childhood malaria. Malaria depresses the immune system of infected subjects. It is generally accepted that increased mortality in measles – which in West African infants has, at times, been in the region of 30% – is largely a function of poor nutrition. Morley (1969) found that severe measles in West Africa was closely correlated with the incidence of kwashiorkor. In Kenya almost half the deaths from measles in the Kenyatta National Hospital occurred in nutritionally deficient children under the age of 1 year (Alwar, 1992). Elsewhere, it was shown that supplementation of patients deficient in vitamin A could reduce the mortality from measles by at least 50%; and it was calculated that supplementation of all deficient children worldwide would prevent between one and three million deaths a year (Sommer, 1993).

It might be thought that ecological factors have a material role only or mainly in zoonotic infections. That this is not so is shown by the foregoing examples of the influence of malnutrition on the outcome of infection. It can also be demonstrated by two rather different historical excursions. In Britain in the earlier part of the nineteenth century working-class people were generally poor. Poverty, bad housing, overcrowding and malnutrition were so common as to be the norm among quite large parts of the population. Under such conditions measles was an extremely serious disease of childhood, with case fatality rates in the region of 5%, compared with a rate of about 0.02% in Britain after the Second World War, but before the advent of effective vaccination – a 250-fold difference.

In the absence of vaccination programmes epidemic outbreaks of measles in developed countries tend to occur at intervals of 3 years or so, affecting (mainly) school children of 5–10 or 12 years of age. The younger ages are more heavily involved because most of the older children will have acquired immunity from earlier outbreaks. Preschool children at home tend to be protected from exposure to the aerosols of virus which spread infection among groups, but are, of course, exposed to the virus which infected older siblings might bring home.

In developing countries, with very different habitats and social interactions the ecology of human populations is clearly different from that in developed countries. Very young children, for example, tend to be carried about outside the home much more, where they are correspondingly more likely to be exposed to infection at an early age. Case fatality rates for measles are highest in the very young and the old – circumstances demonstrable at very different levels of mortality in both settled endemic and virgin-soil situations (Christensen et al., 1952; Celers, 1965). In the Greenland outbreak analysed by Christensen and colleagues (1952), the virus was brought into the country by a young Greenlander returning from Denmark while incubating the infection. The disease occurred predominantly in three urban settlements, where the morbidity reached 99.9% of a population of 4320. Forty-five per cent of the patients suffered complications – mainly pneumonia, there were six cases of encephalitis with four deaths. Eighty-three pregnant women were infected, of whom seven aborted between the third and fifth months. Two full-term infants died within 24 hours of birth, and three of six premature infants died. The overall death rate in the outbreak was 18 per 1000. In low-density populations infectious cases of the disease have a smaller likelihood of infecting others than in high-density populations – a further example of the influence of ecology on epidemiology. Conversely, the duration of an epidemic outbreak is lengthened in the presence of low population density – with the proviso that in an extremely dispersed population index cases may well have become non-infectious by the time they make contact with further susceptibles.

After an incubation period of 10–12 days in children (but longer in older subjects), there is a prodromal period of 2 or 3 days during which the patient is feverish and virus is present in nasal secretions, tears, the throat and the urine; this last being an indication of the widespread dissemination and multiplication of the virus in the infected body. Towards the end of the prodromal period spots (Koplik spots) appear in the mucous membranes of the mouth and pharynx. The Koplik spots are followed by the appearance of the rash in the skin, and very rapidly by antibody in the blood. Soon after the appearance of the antibody the virus is cleared from the body; the patient, although no longer infectious, may continue to feel ill for a few days. Deaths from measles may result from direct action of the virus in causing a pneumonia, or it may be due to secondary bacterial infection facilitated by a depression of immunity late in incubation and during the prodromal period. Recovery from measles is accompanied by immunity which is solid and lifelong.

About one patient in 200 has a brief fit during the feverish period of the infection. Recovery from such fits is virtually complete. However, about one in 2000 develops encephalitis; the incidence is two or three times greater in children over the age of 10 than it is in those younger than 5. Case fatality rates of measles encephalitis vary between 10 and 15%, and roughly a quarter of the survivors suffer some degree of brain damage. A rare, slowly progressive, and eventually fatal, neurological disease – subacute sclerosing panencephalitis (SSPE) – is occasionally diagnosed in school children who generally have had measles several years earlier, about half of them before they were 2 years old. SSPE, like measles itself and measles encephalitis can be prevented by timely immunization with potent measles vaccine.

Because SSPE has its greatest incidence in children who were infected in infancy, measles vaccination is best done before the age of 1 year, preferably after the infant's sixth month. Until that time, maternally transmitted passive immunity to measles is likely to interfere with the efficacy of the vaccine. Infants and children in developed and many developing countries are subjected to a rather large number of immunizations which are frequently offered as components of a vaccine cocktail. If a baby can be given three or four of the necessary immunizations at a time, the number of visits to the clinic can be sensibly reduced. MMR vaccine (mentioned above) is clearly an advance on previously available vaccines – not least because its early use in all (or almost all) babies ensures the likelihood of a high degree of herd immunity against infection by rubella virus (see below).

An unlooked for result of vaccination programmes which fail to immunize virtually all the susceptible children by the time they transfer from primary to secondary school is that groups of adolescents and young adults with no, or inadequate, immunity are liable to be infected, when the disease is more severe than it would have been at a much earlier age. The frequency of this hazard will increase if vaccination programmes are not continued vigorously enough after their introduction. The disease in adults is more severe than it is in otherwise healthy First World children. In the eighteenth and nineteenth centuries, when European and American explorers and whale hunters were voyaging in the Pacific Ocean, they introduced measles into several island communities which had never before experienced it. The results were reported as catastrophic, with high morbidity and mortality, accompanied by severe disruption of the affected societies. There is no reason to doubt these accounts, but epidemic statistics for these outbreaks are, unfortunately, lacking. The first well-documented account of a so-called virgin soil epidemic relates to the introduction of measles into Greenland in 1951, discussed above. In a population of more than 4000 – confined to a few coastal communities – only five people were not infected within a period of 6 weeks (Christensen et al., 1952).

Even in well-conducted programmes about 10% of vaccinated children either fail to respond or respond inadequately (Lerman et al., 1993; Ramsay et al., 1994). These cohorts of susceptibles will eventually become groups of adolescents or young adults among whom it will be possible for the measles virus to circulate. The greatest danger of death is faced by those under the age of 1 year and above the age of 10 years when they are infected by the measles virus. In one study, the death rate in those older than 15 was almost 90 per 100 000. To avoid this sort of outcome it appears from a study of a measles outbreak on a university campus that a successful vaccination rate of more than 98% may be needed (Allen et al., 1993), and that immunization is not always effective in children. Whether this is due to failures of vaccine or to other causes is unclear, but although there had been no change in vaccine coverage among preschool children, and no apparent change in the previously high vaccine efficacy, there was a sharp increase, of more than fourfold, in measles incidence in the USA in 1989–90 (King et al., 1991; Gindler et al., 1992).

Eradication of an infectious disease implies the complete, global absence of the disease and the causal pathogen. Smallpox is the only disease which has so far been eradicated. Elimination implies the removal of the disease and its causal agent from an individual country or region. The findings mentioned above introduce some important doubts about the possibility of eradicating measles; and even elimination may be difficult to achieve.

Quite clearly, if immunization is to alter the ecological relationship between measles virus and humankind, it must be done very thoroughly and consistently from generation to generation in a large enough proportion of the susceptible population to ensure the induction of herd immunity. This would, of course, carry with it the possibility of breaking the transmission of the virus and thus eliminating the disease. But it would remain eliminated only as long as the herd immunity was maintained by regular vaccination and revaccination, since 'a one dose strategy has not eliminated measles in any country despite high coverage' (Cutts and Markowitz, 1994), an opinion subsequently confirmed by observations in the Gambia (Mulholland, 1995). Its elimination depends also on the absence of scattered small reservoirs of infection in nomadic populations (Loutan and Paillard, 1992). Individual nomadic groups are certainly too small to maintain a permanent circulation of the virus (Black, 1965), but more or less regular meetings of several groups for religious or commercial purposes could give the virus opportunities to move into relatively non-immune populations.

Immunity in response to measles vaccine is not as long lasting as immunity following infection. Young mothers vaccinated in infancy are therefore likely to transfer an inadequate passive immunity to their babies, who may thus be exposed to infection at an age with a relatively high risk of a fatal outcome.

Can measles be eradicated? Measles shares with smallpox the essential attribute which makes it theoretically eradicable: humans are the only known natural host. Since there is no non-human reservoir of the virus, the breaking of transmission wherever measles is endemic, would effectively stop the spread of the virus, and epidemic outbreaks would be a thing of the past. For an eradication programme to be effected – given that the problems of worldwide vaccine supply and delivery could be solved – a simple and quick method of determining the immune status of individuals and communities would be indispensable to ensure that proper coverage had been obtained and vaccine was not being needlessly used to revaccinate already immune subjects. In the smallpox campaign this requirement was met by examining population members superficially for scars of either smallpox or vaccination.

The presence of either signified immunity to smallpox. No such simple method as the scar survey exists for measles; immune status must be assessed by measuring antibody concentration in the blood, or at the very least by determining whether or not a minimum concentration of antibody is present in the blood. Blood samples could rather easily be collected on filter paper after pricking ear lobes or fingers with sterile needles; but the expense and time of laboratory testing would then be necessary. It is, in any case, doubtful that the international community would support such a venture with the same enthusiasm with which the smallpox programme was supported. Measles is not a disease which frightens the citizens of economically well-off countries.

## Mumps

The paramyxovirus causing this painful, but seldom fatal, condition is unrelated to either measles virus or those paramyxoviruses responsible for several respiratory infections. Outbreaks of mumps have been described as *epidemic parotitis*, since the most obvious clinical finding is the painful swelling of the parotid glands which gives the disease its name. The name tends to give a wrong impression of the disease, which may well not be a primary infection of the parotid gland. Naturally occurring mumps is acquired either by inhalation of virus spread in salivary droplets excreted by an infected subject, or by close contact between infected and susceptible subjects. The incubation period is about 18 days, with an infectious period from up to 6 days before to about 4 days after the onset of clinical disease. After direct inoculation of the parotid gland the incubation period is reduced to about a week. This suggests that after infection the virus undergoes replication elsewhere in the body and reaches the salivary glands during a secondary spread.

The virus is always widely disseminated in the body. It has been found not only in the parotid and other salivary glands, but also in the testes, ovaries and pancreas, as well as the thyroid and mammary glands, and in the meninges. It has also been isolated from blood, cerebrospinal fluid, and urine, giving further evidence of the widespread occurrence of the virus in the body. The involvement of the testes, in addition to causing severe pain, may, especially in postpubertal subjects, lead to testicular atrophy, but since this – when it occurs – is generally unilateral, subsequent sterility is not invariable.

Most cases of mumps occur in those aged between 5 and 9 years. This is also the age group in which encephalitis is most common.

Before the widespread use of MMR vaccine, mumps virus was the most frequent cause of encephalitis in Britain and the USA as it probably is in those parts of the world where vaccination is not practised. Although mumps encephalitis almost always clears up completely, there is some evidence that a small proportion of patients may be left with impaired hearing. Immunization in childhood with combined measles, mumps and rubella vaccine, which greatly reduces the incidence of the disease, is therefore to be very strongly recommended.

## Rubella

Also known as German measles, this disease was first recognized and described as a separate entity by German physicians in the seventeenth century. In the mid-nineteenth century the Scot Dr Veale suggested that the condition should be called rubella – and this is what it is widely known as today in the English-speaking world. Infection with the rubella virus is spread by respiratory droplets, causing epidemic disease which is generally quite mild clinically. It may, however, be remarkably destructive and the cause of much personal and familial disturbance.

Rubella is generally considered to be a childhood disease, and is often so mild as to be ignored. The incubation period is between 2 and 3 weeks – the average being about 17 days. Its main features are a mild fever with a sore throat and enlarged glands in the neck. There is usually a rash which often appears and disappears rapidly, especially in children. It consists of separate spots which run together giving the patient a flushed appearance. Some patients may have what seems to be a severe common cold. Adults may have joint pains, mainly in the hips, knees, and ankles. Symptoms seldom last longer than a week, and are not particularly severe; but joint pains, when present, may persist for longer. Other viruses may cause symptoms almost identical with those of rubella. The diseases they cause are generally not particularly serious and failure to make a correct diagnosis of rubella is of little importance unless a woman of child-bearing age happens to be exposed to the patient, when the consequences of a mistaken diagnosis can be momentous.

In 1941 Gregg reported from Sydney surprisingly many newborn Australian children with congenital cataracts and other abnormalities of the eye. This phenomenon was not confined to Sydney but was being reported from other parts of Australia as well. When he studied the babies further, Gregg found that many of them also had congenital abnormalities of the heart, and impaired hearing, and – most importantly – that nearly all the mothers had had rubella during the first 3 months of their pregnancies. Despite an initial reluctance to accept that there was a causal relationship between rubella in pregnant women and congenital abnormalities in their infants, during the next 10 years the evidence in favour of Gregg's view accumulated steadily.

In the 1950s in Britain (Manson *et al.*, 1960), Sweden, and the USA (Siegel and Greenberg, 1960), studies on rubella babies showed that when the mother was infected during the first 12 weeks of pregnancy the risk to the baby was of the order of 20% at birth. When the children were re-examined as they got older, and hearing loss could be determined more accurately, the proportion of those with anomalies rose to about 35%. Gregg's triad – as it was called – of abnormalities of the eye, heart, and ear was not always present. As the condition was studied more thoroughly, the Rubella Syndrome, as it came to be called, was more fully defined. The earlier in pregnancy that the mother is infected, the greater is the risk of damage to the fetus. Infection in the first 8–10 weeks of pregnancy leads to damage in up to 90% of fetuses. In subsequent months – up to the fourth – the incidence of damage decreases by about 10% per month. Even after the fourth month damage may be caused, but it is difficult to quantify the risk. Nevertheless, there have been reports of deafness and other abnormalities in children of mothers infected after the fourth month of pregnancy.

The syndrome of congenital rubella infection may continue to develop for many years after the birth of the baby. At birth, in addition to the commonly recognized abnormalities of the heart and defects of the eye, there may be any or all of hepatitis, hepatosplenomegaly, thrombocytopenia, lymphadenopathy, and pathological changes in the bones. As the baby grows, other abnormalities may show themselves, such as chronic diarrhoea, a chronic rash, inadequate development of the thymus gland which leads to inadequacies of immunity, and deficient growth. In childhood, deafness and consequent speech defects may become apparent; growth deficiency becomes more pronounced; the child may develop diabetes mellitus and show signs of thyroid deficiency; and there may be severe disturbances of behaviour. Finally, in adolescence the patient may develop panencephalitis.

In an ordinary, or non-congenital, infection the virus enters the body by the respiratory route and, in the first place, multiplies in the upper respiratory mucous membrane and, probably, the local lymph nodes. This is followed by a viraemia which spreads the virus widely throughout the body. Shedding of virus occurs mainly from the throat and has been detected for a week before the rash appears. Infected subjects may, therefore, be infectious before there is any overt sign of disease. In pregnancy the placenta is infected during the viraemia, and the virus spreads from there to the fetus where it infects cells and destroys them. The earlier in pregnancy that this occurs the more serious is the immediate damage, because cells which would otherwise multiply to form substantial parts of organs disappear, leading to serious deficits in the organs affected. This is especially noticeable in the heart, which may show very severe abnormalities because of the absence of particular groups of cells at crucial stages of its development.

Infants with congenital rubella may excrete the virus for months, and are potential sources of infection for their attendants and others. Such infants carry a wide range of abnormalities. Damage has been found in almost every organ and tissue at one time or another. In addition to the developmental abnormalities caused by cellular deficits, inflammatory changes have been found in the heart and lungs, the middle ear, the liver, the kidney, the eye and the meninges. The damage most frequently seen in congenital rubella is in the heart and the eye, but abnormalities of the blood, the liver, and spleen are common, as are damage to the long bones, and inflammation of the meninges and brain. Deafness and mental handicap of different degrees of severity are common, but are generally noticed later in the development of the child. The involvement of several body systems occurs most often when the fetus is infected in the second month, which is when most of the organs are at critical stages of their development. Such children have a very poor prognosis; many of them die in their first year of life.

In unvaccinated communities rubella, although a disease mainly of young children, also affects adolescents and young adults. A survey in the USA showed that by age 16 about 80% of the population had antibody to rubella virus – indicating previous infection. By the age of 30 about 10% more of those tested had antibody. When epidemic outbreaks of rubella occurred, therefore, they were not confined to the younger age groups, but implicated others, including women of child-bearing age. The disease itself is so trivial that there would be no need to do anything about preventing it, were it not for the very grave risk of a severe outcome in children congenitally infected in the earlier stages of pregnancy.

The most effective way to reduce the risk of congenital rubella is to ensure that women are immune before conception. In the absence of a safe and effective vaccine there is only one way to do this, and that is to ensure that young girls are exposed to natural infection – preferably before the age of puberty. Before suitable vaccines were available, concerned parents would organize 'rubella parties' so that their children – especially the girls – could be exposed to the virus in the home of a friend or acquaintance with an infected child. However, this method of acquiring immunity tended to be rather uncontrolled: mature women could also be infected. In some parts of the world such as the West Indies and Hawaii, even by age 30 only about 40% of the population has specific rubella antibody. Why this should be is not understood. Clearly, epidemic outbreaks of the disease in such circumstances could lead to a devastatingly high incidence of babies with congenital abnormalities.

The best way of preventing congenital rubella and all the emotional disturbance, financial hardship, and economic cost that it brings with it is to vaccinate the population at risk. Rubella vaccines consist of live, attenuated virus, i.e. they infect the recipients. The choice of vaccine strain is important. The one used in Great Britain is capable of causing some of the symptoms of the naturally acquired disease, but also confers an enduring immunity. There are two main policies for vaccinating against rubella. In one – used in Britain until late 1988 – the vaccine is offered to schoolgirls between the ages of 11 and 14, to susceptible women after the birth of their babies, and to women at high occupational risk – teachers, nursery nurses, etc. Vaccination of enough school-girls will eventually provide highly immune child-bearing cohorts, but the amount of virus present in the community is little reduced because it continues to circulate among boys and younger girls. The other policy, belatedly adopted in Britain in 1988, aims to immunize all children by the age of 2 to reduce the amount of virus in the community, and thus indirectly to protect susceptible adult females. Vaccine is also given to older girls who have not received the MMR vaccine, and to adults who ask for it. Care must be taken not to vaccinate pregnant women, because there may be a chance that the vaccine virus will induce the congenital rubella syndrome in their fetuses. Susceptible women should be vaccinated either before or after pregnancy. Despite the fact that it uses more vaccine, this is a more cost-effective procedure than the previous one which vaccinated only a relatively small segment of the population at risk, because it not only immunizes the appropriate target group, but also considerably reduces the amount of virus in the environment of potentially pregnant women, and thus the heavy costs involved in caring for children damaged *in utero*.

# References

Allen, L. J., Lewis, T., Martin, C. F. *et al.* (1993). Analysis of a measles epidemic. *Statistical Medicine* **12**, 229–239.

Alwar, A.J.E. (1992). The effect of protein energy malnutrition on morbidity and mortality due to measles at Kenyatta National Hospital. *East African Medical Journal* **69**, 415–418.

Black, F.L. (1965). Measles endemicity in insular populations: critical community size and its evolutionary implication. *Theoretical Biology* **11**, 207–211.

Black, F.L., Hierholzer, W., Woodall, J.P. and Pinheiro, F. (1971). Intensified ractions to measles vaccine in unexposed populations of American Indians. *Journal of Infectious Diseases* **124**, 306–317.

Celers, J. (1965). Problèmes de santé publique posés par la rougeole dans les pays favorisés. *Archiv fur der gesamte Virusforschung* **16**, 5–18.

Christensen, P.R., Henning, S., Bang, H.O. *et al.* (1952). An epidemic of measles in southern Greenland, 1951: measles in virgin soil. II The epidemic proper. *Acta Medica Scandinavica* **144**, 430–449.

Cutts, F.R. and Markowitz, L.E. (1994). Successes and failures in measles control. *Journal of Infectious Diseases* **170**, (Suppl.1), S31–S41.

Gindler, J.S., Atkinson, W.L., Markowitz, L.E. and Hutchins, S.S. (1992). Epidemiology of measles in the United States in 1989 and 1990. *Pediatric Infectious Diseases Journal* **11**, 841–846.

Gregg, N.M. (1941). Congenital cataract following German measles in the mother. *Transactions of the Ophthalmological Society of Australia* **3**, 35–46.

King, G.E., Markowitz, L.E., Patriarca, P.A. and Dales, L.G. (1991). The clinical efficacy of measles vaccine during the 1990 measles epidemic. *Pediatric Infectious Diseases Journal* **10**, 883–887.

Lerman, Y., Riskin-Mashiach, S., Cohen, D. *et al.* (1993). Immunity to measles in young adults in Israel. *Infection* **21**, 154–157.

Loutan, L. and Paillard, S. (1992). Measles in a West African nomadic community. *Bulletin of the World Health Organization* **70**, 741–744.

Manson, M.M., Logan, P.D. and Loy, R.M. (1960). Rubella and other virus infections during pregnancy. *Report on Public Health and Medical Subjects*, no. 101, Her Majesty's Stationery Office, London.

Morley, D. (1969). The severe measles of West Africa. *Proceedings of the Royal Society of Medicine* **57**, 846–849.

Mulholland, K. (1995). Measles and pertussis in developing countries with good vaccine coverage. *Lancet* **345**, 305–307.

Neel, J.V., Centerwall, W.R., Chagnon, N.A. and Casey, H.L. (1970). Notes on the effect of measles in virgin-soil population of South American Indians. *American Journal of Epidemiology* **91**, 418–429.

Ramsay, M., Gay, N., Miller, E. *et al.* (1994). The epidemiology of measles in England and Wales: rationale for the 1994 national vaccination campaign. *Communicable Disease Report* **4**, R141–R146.

Siegel, M. and Greenberg, M. (1960). Fetal death, malformation and prematurity after maternal rubella: results of prospective study, 1949–1958. *New England Journal of Medicine* **262**, 389–393.

Sommer, A. (1993). Vitamin A, infectious disease, and childhood mortality: a solution? *Journal of Infectious Diseases* **167**, 1003–1007.

# Chapter 4

# Influenza

The classical symptoms of epidemic influenza – cough, aching muscles, shivering, and sweating – appear in many ancient descriptions of diseases. Some of the conditions may, in fact, have been influenza as we know it, but even as late as the Elizabethan and early Stuart periods the English sweats (probably influenza) had not been disentangled from other clinical conditions in which fever and sweating occurred. 'Influenza' is the Italian word which was used in the fourteenth or fifteenth centuries to explain the origin of the disease, which was believed to result from the influence of 'unusual conjunctions of planets at times of epidemics of coughs, colds and fever' (Stuart-Harris and Schild, 1976). Thomas Willis, a seventeenth-century medical scientist who described the eponymous arterial circulation at the base of the brain, said that outbreaks of what we can recognize as influenza happened 'as though sent by some blast of the stars'. Some modern, non-medical, scientists appear to believe that epidemic influenza does, indeed, reach the Earth from space; though one may doubt that even experts in astronomy and astrophysics are necessarily qualified in epidemiology.

Most winters in the northern hemisphere see an increase in deaths, especially among the elderly, which are associated with respiratory and cardiac disease (Housworth and Langmuir, 1974). Some of the respiratory disease may be influenza; but to be certain that influenza is the cause of clinically recognizable respiratory disease accompanied by an excess of deaths, clinical diagnoses should be confirmed by isolation and identification of the virus. This is important, because three different types of influenza virus are recognized, known as influenza A, B and C. Antibody studies suggest that influenza C occurs fairly widely, but seems not to be particularly pathogenic. Since there is doubt about whether the virus is, in fact, a member of the influenza group (Melnick, 1971) it will not be considered further. Of the other two, influenza A was isolated first in Great Britain in 1932 (Smith *et al.*, 1933), influenza B 7 or 8 years later in the USA (Francis, 1940). These two viruses cause clinically very similar illnesses, although it is said that type B influenza tends to be milder than type A. Nevertheless, in an outbreak in the USA in 1936 (subsequently identified as type B influenza) the death rate of more than 40 per 100 000 equalled the death rate in the pandemic Asian (type A) influenza of 1957/58. Epidemiologically, however, their behaviour is clearly different, with epidemic outbreaks of influenza A recurring at intervals of, usually, 2–3 years, and epidemic influenza B recurring after 4–7 years.

The two recognizably different forms in which epidemic influenza occurs result from differences in the genomic structures of type A and type B viruses. Both have RNA genomes. In type B viruses the genome consists of a sole piece of single-stranded RNA with its associated protein, while in type A the ribonucleoprotein occurs as eight discrete segments of unequal size. Viruses of each type carry on their surfaces two kinds of spikes. One is the haemagglutinin (HA), a glycoprotein which confers antigenic specificity on the virus; the other, also a glycoprotein, is a neuraminidase (NA) which releases newly replicated virus from the surface of the infected cell. Both glycoproteins undergo antigenic variation, which allows the virus they are part of to escape host neutralizing antibody evoked by the infection. This variation is known as 'antigenic drift' because it occurs more or less continuously, but not precipitously, during outbreaks and the course of non-epidemic infection. Some time after an epidemic outbreak of influenza – usually years, rather than weeks or months – the immunity evoked by that infection is no longer able to protect against infection by the antigenically different virus which has resulted from selection pressure by antibody against the virus which caused the original outbreak. Except for the longer intervals between type B outbreaks, the pattern is similar in both types of infection because both types of virus undergo antigenic drift.

Because of their segmented genome, type A viruses are also subject to a different and more far-reaching antigenic variation than that induced by the drift mechanism. When two virus particles infect the same cell simultaneously the individual pieces of their genomes, after replication, are reassembled pretty well at random, and a full complement of RNA in many, if not most, of the progeny virions will consist of a mixed bag of genetic components. The reassortment may bring antigenically very different HA and NA to the fore. Among this gallimaufry some virions may not be particularly effective, many will be able to operate 'normally', but because the new arrangement of the genome may have caused a major alteration, or 'shift', in antigenicity of HA or NA, or both, the stage would be set for a pandemic outbreak of influenza by a strain of virus against which there is little, if any, pre-existing immunity in the human population of the world. Antigenic shifts occur at intervals; they are movable feasts, with no known method of predicting when the next one will arise. Such pandemic influenza outbreaks are accompanied not only by grossly increased morbidity, but also by increased mortality – especially among those sections of the population at increased risk of death during an 'ordinary' outbreak of the disease. When the antigenicity of HA undergoes a major change a new, and potentially pandemic, strain of influenza A is created. Altered HA and NA are distinguished by numbers, and radically different strains of virus are labelled accordingly. For example, the 1957 Asian (or Singapore) strain of influenza A virus is $A(H_2N_2)$, and the 1968 Hong Kong strain is $A(H_3N_2)$. The HA and NA of animal influenza viruses are indicated appropriately: eq for equine, sw for swine, av for avian. Influenza A viruses contain two internal type-specific antigens, which are the same in all of them, whatever their host provenance. Some of the animal isolates are closely related antigenically to human strains of virus. Shope's strain of swine influenza virus is very similar to the first human strain isolated in 1932. Indeed, it has been suggested that Shope's virus and the 1932 strain were derived by antigenic drift from the strain which caused the pandemic outbreak in 1918. Should a major antigenic shift be accompanied by an enhancement of the virulence of the new strain, the death toll in the subsequent pandemic may be expected to be high – perhaps as high as that of the pandemic of 1918–19, when it was estimated that there were more than 20 000 000 deaths worldwide.

It was believed that the recurrence of epidemic outbreaks of both types of influenza could be predicted – though not with notable precision – because novel antigenic variants seemed to arise 10–15 years after the previous pandemic spread of the disease. However, since the Hong Kong ($H_3N_2$) virus appeared in 1968 (28 years ago, at the time of writing), and 'drifted' variants of it are still current, this belief is clearly without sound foundation. A 'shift' is a rare event which may occur randomly, at any time. Neither the occurrence of a 'new' virus, nor the behaviour of the infection it causes in the subsequent pandemic, can be foretold with any accuracy. Infection rates no doubt depend on the degree of immunity in the population at risk. Since the pandemic strain is, by definition, 'new', all age segments of the population should be equally at risk. However, in the aftermath of the 1957 pandemic caused by the so-called Asian virus, it was found that in a population under attack by the new strain there were a few very old people who were already equipped with antibody specific for the new strain (Mulder and Masurel, 1958). This suggests that previous antigenic configurations may recur. This supposition was confirmed when antibodies against the Hong Kong virus of 1968 were found in sera which had been collected before that virus appeared as the agent of the pandemic of 1968–69 (Davenport *et al.*, 1969). If reassortment produces 'new' strains of virus at random such a view is not unreasonable. In epidemic influenza caused by 'drifted' strains, the highest incidence is to be expected in the younger population segments – those not previously exposed to the virus – typically, 5- to 14-year-olds; with a smaller, but appreciable, incidence in the parental generation of the young people. The overall case fatality rate may vary quite widely from one epidemic outbreak to the next, but those older than 65 years, and sufferers from chronic debilitating conditions such as diseases of the heart and circulation, the respiratory system, the kidneys and diabetes, are at greatest risk of being killed by the infection.

Influenza A viruses tend to be present in populations during interepidemic periods, when they may cause subclinical infections, stimulate immunity, and undergo antigenic drift. The Hong Kong virus ($H_3N_2$) caused two epidemic outbreaks of influenza in Britain in the early days of its circulation. The first, starting towards the end of 1968, was relatively mild, with a low mortality rate. Nevertheless, early in 1969 the virus was distributed widely (Miller *et al.*, 1971), but the epidemic petered out. It recurred at the end of the year and carried over into 1970 with heavy mortality, although there was not a great deal more virus about than there had been after the earlier outbreak. Why this was so is obscure, but the earlier seeding of virus in a population may be a prerequisite for the initiation of an epidemic outbreak. Once the outbreak has begun, however, there is no doubt that the virus is disseminated by the aerial route in aerosols generated by the coughs of infected subjects.

Unlike type B viruses which are confined to humans, type A viruses also occur in a variety of other animals. Natural infection of horses with equine influenza viruses, and pigs with swine influenza viruses occurs commonly, 'the virus' being particularly dreaded by trainers of race horses because of the loss of condition which it causes. Pigs have been found to be naturally susceptible to infection with type A viruses of human origin (Kundin, 1970). Dogs (Nikitin *et al.*, 1972) and cats (Paniker and Nair, 1972) are both susceptible to infection with type A strains, and cats also to type B. After an outbreak of influenza in a human population, antibody specific for the infecting strain was found in 5.6% of serum samples from dogs. In both dogs and cats virus was isolated from nasopharyngeal secretions. It may be that pet animals play a role in epidemic human influenza.

Many different birds are also susceptible to infection with influenza A viruses; however, ducks are a particularly rich source of avian strains of virus. Fowl plague virus and the other influenza viruses of birds and non-human mammals carry haemagglutinins and neuraminadases which are distinct from those found in human viruses, but a reassortment of the genomic fragments made possible by a mixed infection may well produce haemagglutinins and neuraminidases allowing new influenza viruses to infect human beings.

Where the pre-1957 pandemic strains arose is uncertain, but serological studies imply rather strongly that influenza antibodies in people born before 1925 resulted from infection with a virus closely related to Shope's swine virus. Such antibody is absent from those born after 1925, which suggests that the pandemic strain of 1918 carried HA of the same, or very similar, antigenicity as the swine virus. It was generally believed among American pig farmers that their animals went down with swine influenza only after the onset of the human infection, though the origin of that pandemic strain is unknown. There is a strong supposition, however, that both the 1957 ($H_2N_2$) and 1968 ($H_3N_2$) strains originated in South East Asia (Shortridge et al., 1979). The environment of southern China makes it a likely region for the appearance of new pandemic strains (Shortridge and Stuart-Harris, 1984). It is both heavily populated ($> 1000/km^2$) and heavily cultivated. Much of the farming is concerned with the growing of rice, and large flocks of ducks are kept which deal with both insect and shellfish pests in the paddy-fields. In most summers influenza viruses can generally be isolated from agricultural poultry – mainly ducks (including wild ducks), which carry a range of subtypes of influenza A viruses. Influenza viruses, which are excreted from the guts of birds, have been isolated both from faeces on river banks and from lake water. Wildfowl, especially those associated with water, may thus be implicated in the amplification and transmission of new influenza A viruses. Large numbers of pigs are also kept, which probably also play an important part in the generation of 'new' strains of influenza viruses. Human strains of $H_3N_2$ virus are unable to cross the species barrier to infect birds because of incompatibility of the nucleoprotein gene. However, if they undergo re-assortment in pigs the species barrier is crossed more readily because swine strains seem to have a broader host range (Scholtissek et al., 1985). The dense concentration of humans, pigs and waterfowl, especially ducks, thus provides a favourable environment for the appearance and propagation of new strains of influenza A viruses. Admittedly, mixed infection is probably a rare event, even in such a milieu, but so, too, is the emergence of new pandemic strains (Webster and Laver, 1972).

New influenza viruses spread around the world very fast, probably in part by air passengers carrying to distant destinations the virus they are incubating; but an appreciable amount of virus may be carried by migrating birds and far-flying sea birds such as shearwaters and terns which are able to travel great distances with surprising rapidity, and from which influenza viruses have been isolated (Becker, 1963). The general run of influenzal infection can, theoretically, be controlled by vaccination – given that sufficient, and sufficiently potent and non-reactive vaccines become available. However, immunity to influenza A viruses is complicated by the quaintly named 'doctrine of original antigenic sin'. What this means is that the immune response to influenza viruses is conditioned throughout a subject's life by the first strain he or she meets, either by infection or vaccination. Subsequently, contact with influenza A (but not B or C) antigens of strains different from the original one, leads not only to a response to that strain, but also to an anamnestic response to the original strain (Davenport et al., 1953). However, the more purified vaccines available today allow more potent preparations to be used clinically; with them, the specific response to the vaccine strain is at least as good as the anamnestic response to the original antigen(s). Immunization with vaccine containing antigens appropriate to those of the circulating epidemic strain may therefore be expected to produce a significant degree of protection against infection, as long as the virus has not been altered by the antigenic shift mechanism. Given that the correct choice of vaccine antigens has been made, and the vaccine widely enough applied, the worst ravages of 'ordinary' epidemic influenza can probably be contained. But since pandemic influenza – the result of antigenic shift – is pretty certainly zoonotic, there is clearly no prospect of eradicating the infection from the human species.

## References

Becker, W.B. (1963). The morphology of tern virus. *Virology* **20**, 318–327.

Davenport, F.M., Hennessy, A. V. and Francis Jr, T. (1953). Epidemiologic and immunologic significance of age distribution of antibody to antigenic variants of influenza virus. *Journal of Experimental Medicine* **98**, 641–656.

Davenport, F.M., Minuse, E., Hennessy, A.V. and Francis Jr, T. (1969). Interpretation of influenza antibody patterns of man. *Bulletin of the World Health Organization* **41**, 453–460.

Francis Jr, T. (1940). A new type of virus from epidemic influenza. *Science* **92**, 405–408.

Housworth, J. and Langmuir, A.D. (1974). Excess mortality from epidemic influenza, 1957–1966. *American Journal of Epidemiology* **100**, 40–48.

Kundin, W.D. (1970). Hong Kong A2 influenza virus infection among swine during a human epidemic in Taiwan. *Nature* **228**, 857.

Melnick, J.L. (1971). Classification and nomenclature of animal viruses 1971. *Progress in Medical Virology* **13**, 462–484.

Miller, D.L., Pereira, M.S. and Clarke, M. (1971). Epidemiology of the Hong Kong 68 variant of influenza A2 in Britain. *British Medical Journal* **1**, 475–479.

Mulder, J. and Masurel, N. (1958). Pre-epidemic antibody against 1957 strain of Asiatic influenza in serum of older people living in the Netherlands. *Lancet* **i**, 810–814.

Nikitin, T., Cohen, D., Todd, J.D. and Lief, F.S. (1972). Epidemiological studies of A/Hong Kong/68 virus infection in dogs. *Bulletin of the World Health Organization* **47**, 471–479.

Paniker, K.J. and Nair, C.M.G. (1972). Experimental infection of animals with influenza-virus types A and B. *Bulletin of the World Health Organization* **47**, 461–463.

Scholtissek, C., Bünger, H., Kistner, O. and Shortridge, K.F. (1985). The nucleoprotein as a possible major factor in determining host specificity of influenza $H_3N_2$ viruses. *Virology* **147**, 287–294.

Smith, W., Andrewes, C.H. and Laidlaw, P.P. (1933). A virus obtained from influenza patients. *Lancet* **ii**, 66–68.

Shortridge, K.F. and Stuart-Harris, C.H. (1984). An influenza epicentre? *Lancet* **ii**, 812–813.

Shortridge, K.F., Butterfield, W.K., Webster, R.G. and Campbell, C.H. (1979). Diversity of influenza A subtypes isolated from domestic poultry in Hong Kong. *Bulletin of the World Health Organization* **57**, 465–469.

Stuart-Harris, C.H. and Schild, G.C. (1976). *Influenza: The Viruses and the Disease*. Edward Arnold, London.

Webster, R.G. and Laver, W.G. (1972). The origin of pandemic influenza. *Bulletin of the World Health Organization* **47**, 449–452.

# Chapter 5

# Tuberculosis

This ancient disease – characterized in 1680 by John Bunyan as 'the Captain of all these Men of Death' – has by no means been vanquished, although mortality rates and incidence in the western world have decreased steadily for almost 150 years. In 1851 the death rate from pulmonary tuberculosis in England and Wales was almost 290 per 100 000; immediately before the Second World War it was less than 50 per 100 000. The decline continued for about 40 years after the war, but stopped in the later years of the 1980s. In many other developed countries the long-continued decreasing incidence of the disease has either been stabilized or reversed. In the USA there were 28 000 more cases between 1985 and 1990 than were expected on the basis of the figures for the previous 30 years. Between 1987 and 1990 in the USA, clinical tuberculosis in children younger than 5 years increased by 39% (Starke *et al.*, 1992), and in 1990 there were more than 25 000 new cases of clinical tuberculosis in both adults and children. Although much of the 'new' tuberculosis in the USA is associated with the AIDS epidemic, it is still in large part a disease of the poor and indigent – in short, a disease of the under class, from which, however, the better off are not exempt.

In Britain, between 1988 and 1993, about 8000 more cases of tuberculosis were notified than would have been expected had the trend of earlier years continued (Hayward and Watson, 1995). In 1982 about one-fifth of the reported cases were non-respiratory tuberculosis; in 1993 more than a quarter were. Not unexpectedly, there was more tuberculosis in large conurbations than in rural areas. Although there was, in general, a higher incidence in immigrants from the Indian subcontinent, this was not so in Bradford and Leicester, which probably have the largest, but also the most firmly established, Asian communities in Britain. This adds a certain weight to the view that among the many factors promoting the spread of tuberculosis, that of unsettled social circumstances is, indeed, important.

In developing countries it remains the prime cause of disease and death. According to the World Health Organization tuberculosis is the most widely prevalent disease in the world. The available figures of incidence are not precise, but between a quarter and a third of the world's population are infected, although some estimates put the proportion as high as a half. The vast majority of infections are latent; but under suitably depressed socioeconomic conditions – however caused – such infections are liable to be reactivated. Despite the fact that only about 5% of those infected fail to develop enough immunity to overcome the infection, there are between eight and ten million new cases of clinical tuberculosis and between three and five million deaths from the disease each year. It kills more adults than any other disease, and is still the Captain of all these Men of Death.

With the success, from the late 1940s and the 1950s onwards, of chemotherapy for this debilitating and fatal disease, much of the mechanism for finding cases and their contacts in the countries of the developed world was allowed to decay because of the belief that the disease was (or soon would be) conquered. Indeed, the combination of pharmacological treatment of infected people, a generally improved standard of living and vaccination of children with BCG, led to a spectacular diminution in the incidence of tuberculosis in Western Europe, North America, and elsewhere among those population segments which enjoyed similar high living standards. Because of this steady reduction in its incidence, tuberculosis was regarded as a disease of diminishing public-health importance, and health department budgets for its control were reduced. When public-health policy was reformulated in this way, no account seems to have been taken of the pathology of tuberculosis, the genetics of microbial resistance to antibiotics, or the compliance of patients in persevering with their medication over periods of many months.

The aetiology of tuberculosis is complex. The microorganism responsible for the lesions which occur during the course of the illness is *Mycobacterium tuberculosis*, but infection with it, although necessary for the development of clinical symptoms, is not, of itself, a sufficient cause of disease. Transmission is overwhelmingly by the respiratory route, and pulmonary tuberculosis is, beyond doubt, the most significant clinical manifestation in the epidemiology of the disease. Infection by other mycobacteria – *M. bovis* and the saprophytic, sometimes falcultatively parasitic, mycobacteria – often occurs by other routes. *M. bovis*, present in the milk of tuberculous cows, is ingested by mouth, causing intestinal tuberculosis and also tuberculosis of bones and joints. Infection by *M. bovis* is rare in developed countries today, largely because bovine tuberculosis is strictly controlled, and milk is almost universally pasteurized, but it still occurs in Third World countries. The saprophytes may be acquired by ingestion or by their contact with injured skin. However acquired, when these infections cause disease it tends, like tuberculosis, to be chronic. Tuberculous infection of other organs and tissues, including, bone, kidneys, lymph nodes, the meninges and many others, also occurs, and is often extremely harmful to the sufferer, but is of less significance than the pulmonary form in disseminating the infection.

Among the more important factors which determine whether or not infected persons will develop tuberculous disease are the size of the infecting dose, and their age, general state of health, economic status and ethnic origin. The very young, especially children younger than 5, are at high risk. Malnutrition, debilitating illness, depressed immunity, alcoholism, metabolic diseases – especially diabetes mellitus – all predispose to the development of tuberculous disease. The poor, being less able to afford a good standard of uncrowded housing, to keep themselves warm enough in winter, and to buy enough of the right kinds of food, as a social class have less resistance to infection than the wealthier strata of society. Ethnic origin is a clear predisposing factor among the Inuit people of Greenland and the far north of Canada, among Amazonian tribes, and among the blacks of South Africa. The Inuit and Amerinds have only recently been exposed to the tubercle bacillus in the remote areas in which they live. The pressure of disease has clearly not had time to select for increased resistance in these populations. In southern Africa the Khoi Khoi (or Hottentots) made contact with the tubercle bacillus (and smallpox virus, among others) when whites from the Netherlands began the occupation of the Cape of Good Hope in 1652. Tuberculosis and smallpox between them destroyed large numbers of Khoi Khoi; other white men's diseases, such as syphilis and alcohol, ensured the disintegration of their society. The Bantu met tuberculosis when they came into contact with the whites in the eighteenth century, but met it in force from about 1880 when the diamond and gold mines and, subsequently, industry, needed the labour of very large numbers of them. The Europeans who introduced the infection to these people had been exposed for many generations to the tubercle bacillus, and it is not unreasonable to assume that populations with a degree of resistance have been selected by an evolutionary process not unlike that which has produced races of rabbits resistant to myxomatosis. Population groups only recently in contact with tubercle bacilli would thus be pretty well fully susceptible, as shown by the high incidence of rapidly fatal, often miliary, tuberculosis to which South

African blacks of all ages are liable. In addition to this probably genetically determined susceptibility, the blacks, uprooted from the comparative plenty of their traditional rural life, were introduced on the mines and in the towns, to urban poverty, and often squalor, overcrowding, and malnutrition – all important factors in ensuring the rapid epidemic spread of any infection, especially tuberculosis. Other, politico-economic, factors saw them crowded into small, hilly areas of the country, not very suitable for agriculture. A high proportion of the men spent most of the year working as labourers in industry and the mines, where they were exposed to tuberculous and venereal infections which they took back to the so-called Native Reserves where the diseases spread freely.

In all forms of tuberculosis the typical lesion develops in much the same way. The first reaction to the presence of tubercle bacilli in a tissue is a brief acute inflammatory response in which infiltrating neutrophils are destroyed by the mycobacteria. This is followed by the infiltration of macrophages derived from circulating blood monocytes. The bacteria are very soon taken up by the macrophages which undergo a change in appearance: with pale cytoplasm and elongated nuclei they resemble (but are not) epithelial cells, and hence are known as *epithelioid* cells. Some of the macrophages fuse, forming large cells with peripherally placed nuclei – the *Langhans giant cells*. This mass of altered macrophages is surrounded by a zone of lymphocytes and fibroblasts. Within about 14 days the centre of this cell mass, consisting of altered macrophages, cells of the invaded tissue and mycobacteria, undergoes coagulative necrosis which, perhaps because of its high lipid content, resists autolysis, and is described as caseous because of its cheese-like appearance. With its caseous centre this cell mass is now a tuberculous follicle or granuloma. The granulomatous tissue typical of tuberculous lesions is constituted by a collection of follicles. The follicle develops before the appearance of detectable immunity, and is a significant, but non-specific, defence response of the infected subject. The caseation is induced mainly by hypersensitivity to tuberculoprotein and other products of the mycobacteria, and therefore depends on their continued multiplication. However, ischaemia is also involved because the peripherally situated blood supply of the granuloma is insufficient to support the large number of infiltrated cells.

At this early stage the granuloma tends to limit the spread of the infection, and if immunity rather than hypersensitivity is well developed, the outcome may be complete resolution, or the lesion may heal and be enclosed in a dense fibrous network, with subsequent slow calcification of the caseous material. The mycobacteria within the healed tubercle may, at any time in the future, resume their pathogenic activity if failing immunity permits the breakdown of the fibrous barrier and the activation of the bacteria.

When hypersensitivity is in the ascendant, active caseous tuberculosis results. The tubercles enlarge and multiply and the disease progresses with considerable destruction of tissue. The caseous material softens and liquifies, and in the lung this leads to the formation of cavities and not infrequently the erosion of blood vessels, causing the patient to produce blood-stained or frankly bloody sputum containing many mycobacteria which will usually be disseminated in the environment, unless care is taken to cover coughs and dispose carefully of sputum and any objects contaminated by it. Liquified caseous material is all to likely to enter a large bronchus because its wall has been eroded, allowing the contents of the cavity to drain into it. This leads to widespread caseous bronchopneumonia, with possible spread of infection to whole lobes of the lung. Should there be a strong hypersensitivity reaction very severe systemic effects follow, leading quite swiftly to the death of the patient – but not before he or she has excreted innumerable bacteria in pulmonary droplets.

A third possibility is the development of non-reactive tuberculosis. In this condition the tuberculin reaction – an indicator of infection with *M. tuberculosis*, but not necessarily of disease – is absent. There are masses of bacteria, and much caseation, but no cellular reaction. The outlook for the patient and also for his or her immediate environment is grave. This type of disease is seen in immune deficiency states, as a complication of bone-marrow disease such as leukaemia, and sometimes in the elderly in whom immunity may fail as part of the ageing process. Antituberculous immunity is largely cellular, depending on the activity of macrophages and lymphocytes.

Governments have now accepted the views of the scientists of the Intergovernmental Panel on Climate Change that the world is in the process of global warming because of increasing atmospheric concentrations of the so-called greenhouse gases – especially carbon dioxide, water vapour and methane (Houghton *et al.*, 1995). The problem will be compounded by the reduction of stratospheric ozone, since this will permit the entry into the atmosphere of increased amounts of ultraviolet (UV) radiation. The UVB and UVC components of the ultraviolet are potentially very damaging; DNA and aromatic proteins absorb large amounts of each. UVB not only disrupts DNA, but has wide reaching effects on the immune-system cells in the skin. The changes include an increase in the number of suppressor T cells, and a reduction in the number of circulating helper T cells (Hersey et al., 1983). In patients with tuberculosis this would clearly be very deleterious, and liable to increase the number of sputum-positive individuals spreading their infection. These effects of increased irradiation by UBV would not, of course, be confined to tuberculosis. The reduction in activity of the immune system induced by such increased radiation could well have a significant effect in countries – especially tropical countries – with a low standard of living and and a considerable prevalence of infectious diseases (Leaf, 1989). There is also some evidence that immunity may be related to the cycle of solar activity. Circulating immunoglobulin concentrations were found to be lowest at the peak of solar activity, and increased as the number of sunspots diminished (Stoubel et al., 1995). The effects on the immune system of the two factors could be additive during periods of increased solar activity.

In the United States much of the observed increase in tuberculosis has occurred in people infected with the human immunodeficiency virus (HIV), and a considerable amount of it results from the reactivation of the bacteria in a previously healed lesion. In subjects with immune deficiency, miliary tuberculosis is common.

In the developed countries the changing incidence of tuberculosis has been related to, but not necessarily caused by, increased immigration from the Third World. In Britain ethnic origin is not routinely recorded in epidemiological data, but special surveys have shown that the incidence of the disease is greater in persons of Indian and Pakistani origin than in either the indigenous Caucasian population, or in Afro-Caribbeans (Blair and Balfour, 1993). As was pointed out above, the increase in tuberculosis has not been noted in the well-established and stable Asian communities of Bradford and Leicester; it may, however, be related to the undoubted increase in poverty and homelessness in Britain between about 1980 and the mid-1990s.

The more heavily endemic a region is for tuberculosis, the earlier in life are people infected, and the greater the death rate in children. Not everyone who is infected inevitably develops the disease. Some people – the proportion is higher in those countries and social classes with high living standards – manage to overcome the initial infection and, quite literally, wall it off. A calcified focus can be seen in the chest X-rays of these people. However, if the individual's resistance is reduced for any reason, such as malnutrition, substandard housing, intercurrent infection, old age or suppression of immunity, the walled-off tubercle bacilli are liable to break out of their captivity and reactivate the disease. In countries like Great Britain and the USA this is a very likely way for an elderly relative such as a grandparent – infected in childhood with subsequent healing – to become an excreter of mycobacteria and put the grandchildren at risk of infection.

With the advent of antibiotics in the late 1940s and onwards – half a century ago at the time of writing – it became possible to treat tuberculosis actively with a high probability of success. Chest hospitals and tuberculosis sanatoria in economically developed countries quite rapidly became redundant. At the same time BCG vaccine – a preparation of attenuated bovine tubercle bacilli – was increasingly used to immunize school children and other high-risk groups. The incidence of tuberculosis declined precipitously and the case finding and other measures necessary to keep the disease in check were disbanded or allowed to decay. Tuberculosis is now more prevalent worldwide than it has ever been. Some of those involved in measures to prevent the disease believe that when the risk of infection is sufficiently reduced, the vaccination of school children can be discontinued. However, because of the slowing – and in some places reversal – of the reduction in the incidence of the disease, it would be unsafe to assume that the risk is now reduced (or about to be reduced) sufficiently; nor is it likely to be reduced in the foreseeable future.

Soon after the introduction of effective pharmacological treatment of tuberculosis it was realized that strains of tubercle bacilli resistant to treatment were appearing because of irregular dosage or non-compliance by patients. Unfortunately, this happens all too frequently, and not only in Third World countries. Drug resistance can be avoided by treating patients with several different antibiotics simultaneously; but non-compliance now leads to the appearance of multiple resistance to the commonly used drugs. This makes the management of open tuberculosis more difficult and more expensive than it might be, since the way to ensure compliance by patients is to supervise their drug taking at the prescribed times. However, the effectiveness even of this approach to therapy cannot be relied upon for success when the patient is infected by a strain of *M. tuberculosis* exhibiting multiple resistance to therapeutic agents. Even in the most favourable circumstances the tubercle bacillus is a very persistent pathogen that is not easy to control.

There are several possible reasons for the undoubted increase in tuberculosis in some countries of the developed world. Introduction by immigration from the Third World has been mentioned. Such introduction is likely to increase if the pressure of immigration increases from overpopulated countries subjected to increasingly frequent periods of drought, which is among the predicted consequences of climatic change. Another is increasing immune deficit in people of light skin colour, which will result from increased exposure to sunlight and enhanced amounts of UVB. Malaria tends to depress immunity. If its range increases because climatic change expands the potential habitats of anopheline mosquitoes (among others), this too could increase the number of people with deficient immunity, and thus the incidence of reactivated tuberculosis. Some tuberculosis is already related to immunosuppressive medicines given for the treatment of particular diseases, some by drug addiction, but an increasing amount by infection with HIV.

Immunity reduced by HIV allows latent tuberculous infection to be reactivated and to spread rapidly in the lungs and also to other parts of the body. This can be seen happening in much of Africa, where the incidence of tuberculosis, infection with HIV, and AIDS are high. There are some who believe that little, if anything, can be done to reverse this state of affairs, but this view is not universal (Stanford *et al.*, 1991). People infected with HIV who do not have latent tuberculosis also have no immunity to it and cannot make a suitable immune response to infection. They are thus highly susceptible to the disease. The epidemic spread of AIDS is thus being accompanied in large areas of Africa and parts of the USA by epidemic pulmonary tuberculosis, although the epidemiology of tuberculosis is not yet (in 1996) significantly linked with AIDS in Great Britain. In the Third World the medical and public-health services are unable to do much to contain these destructive epidemic diseases.

This prospective increase in tuberculosis may well be compounded by an increasing incidence of drug-resistant strains of *M. tuberculosis*. In the 10-year period 1982–1991, out of more than 16 000 isolates of tubercle bacilli in England and Wales, more than 1800 (i.e. at least 11%) were found to be resistant to at least one of the most frequently used antituberculous drugs (Warburton *et al.*, 1993). Experience in countries with a greater incidence of drug-resistant strains indicates that treatment of tuberculosis with antibiotics must be closely supervised to ensure that patients take full doses of their medicines and complete their treatments, so that as few resistant strains of bacteria as possible appear.

Since *M. tuberculosis* is an intracellular parasite, immunity to it is mainly cell mediated. Lymphokines produced by sensitized T cells activate macrophages which are the effector cells. The response depends on which populations of T cells are involved, because macrophages respond differently to T cells of different specificity. If T cells specific for certain protein antigens, especially tuberculo-protein, are implicated, then delayed hypersensitivity will result. Circulating T cells and macrophages which are recruited into the resulting acute local inflammatory response are activated and are probably responsible for much of the tissue destruction which characterizes tuberculosis.

There is no correlation between delayed hypersensitivity and immunity in tuberculosis. The tuberculin response – an intradermal delayed hypersensitivity reaction – is used to detect infected individuals in surveys of the incidence of infection. Although the test has been used for many years, and the reagents are now highly purified and reasonably uniform, responses in different countries are not necessarily comparable, not only because of differences in testing techniques, but also because of infection by mycobacteria other than *M. tuberculosis*. In developed countries, *M. bovis*, in the first half of the twentieth century a frequent cause of tuberculous infection, has been largely eliminated by a combination of pasteurization of milk, and the eradication of bovine tuberculosis by regular tuberculin testing of herds and the rigorous exclusion of positively reacting cattle. Other mycobacteria, mostly saprophytic, are capable of causing opportunistic infections with very similar pathology to that of tuberculosis in patients with some predisposing condition. Some of these environmental mycobacteria, however, are able to cause disease in apparently healthy subjects. Non-tuberculous mycobacteria cause a small but pretty steady incidence of disease. Despite the complication they offer, in the hands of competent individuals the results of tuberculin-test surveys can be extremely useful to health authorities; but it must be remembered that although a positive test implies infection, it does not necessarily indicate disease.

Modulating the immune response to *M. tuberculosis* towards immunity instead of hypersensitivity might make treatment with antituberculous drugs more effective in a shorter time, with non-compliance becoming a less significant bar to the rapid attainment of a non-infective state with a consequent reduction in the amount of circulating *M. tuberculosis*. Stanford and colleagues (Bahr *et al.*, 1990; Stanford *et al.*, 1990) claimed that patients immunized with various killed preparations of the saprophyte *M. vaccae* after the start of chemotherapy had improved immune responses to *M. tuberculosis* and, with at least one preparation, there was improved resolution of cavities 3 months after the immunization. The immunity offered may be valuable in dealing with small numbers of drug-resistant bacteria at an early stage of treatment, thus reducing the likelihood of transmission. In a different approach to the problem, mice immunized with DNA vaccines encoding genes for different mycobacterial antigens (Huygen *et al.*, 1996; Tascon *et al.*, 1996) were protected against challenge by *M. tuberculosis*.

Developments on these lines may well lead to vaccines able to stimulate protective immunity more effectively than BCG vaccine.

# References

Bahr, G.M., Shabaan, M.A., Gabriel, M. *et al.* (1990). Improved immunotherapy for pulmonary tuberculosis with *Mycobacterium vaccae*. *Tubercle* **71**, 259–266.

Blair, I. and Balfour, P. (1993). Tuberculosis in the West Midlands, 1990–1991. *Communicable Disease Report* **3**, R154–R157.

Hayward, A.C. and Watson, J.M. (1995). Tuberculosis in England and Wales 1982–1993: notifications exceed predictions. *Communicable Disease Reports* **3**, R29–R33.

Hersey, P., Haran, G., Hasic, E. and Edwards, A. (1983). Alteration of T cell subsets and induction of suppressor T cell activity in normal subjects after exposure to sunlight. *Journal of Immunology* **131**, 171–174.

Houghton, J.T., Meirofilho, L.G., Callander, B.A. *et al.* (eds) (1995). *Climate Change 1995. The Science of Climate Change.* Contributions of Work Group 1 for IPCC. Cambridge University Press, Cambridge.

Huygen, K., Content, J., Denis, O. *et al.* (1996). Immunogenicity and protective efficacy of a tuberculosis DNA vaccine. *Nature Medicine* **2**, 893–898.

Leaf, A. (1989). The potential health effects of global climatic and environmental change. *New England Journal of Medicine* **321**, 1577–1583.

Stanford, J.L., Bahr, G.M., Rook, G.A.W. *et al.* (1990). Immunotherapy with *Mycobacterium vaccae* as an adjunct to chemotherapy in the treatment of pulmonary tuberculosis. *Tubercle* **71**, 87–93.

Stanford, J.L., Grange, J.M. and Pozniak, A. (1991). Is Africa lost? *Lancet* **338**, 557–558.

Starke, J.R., Jacobs, R.F. and Jereb, I. (1992). Resurgence of tuberculosis in children. *Journal of Pediatrics* **120**, 839–855.

Stoubel, E.G., Abramson, E., Gabbay, U. and Pick, A.I. (1995). Relationship between immunoglobulin levels and extremes of solar activity. *International Journal of Biometeorology* **38**, 88–91.

Tascon, R.E., Colston, M.J., Ragno, S. *et al.* (1996). Vaccination against tuberculosis by DNA vaccine. *Nature Medicine* **2**, 888–892.

Warburton, A.R.E., Jenkins, P.A., Waight, P.A. and Watson, J.M. (1993). Drug resistance in initial isolates of *Mycobacterium tuberculosis* in England and Wales, 1982–1991. *Communicable Disease Report* **3**, R175–R179.

# Chapter 6

# Sexually transmitted infections

Sexually transmitted diseases are found in every part of the world. They are clinically diverse, with causative agents spanning a range of unrelated microorganisms including bacteria, mycoplasmas, and viruses. The aetiologies of these diseases are also diverse, but all share a common transmission mechanism – sexual, usually copulatory, activity. They cause few acute deaths. Some – the bacterial infections – can, with timely diagnosis and treatment, be cured; but in the absence of adequate treatment they become chronic, causing an immense amount of illness and debility. When patients with such chronic diseases do eventually die, they do so after suffering much distress – social, physical and mental.

These diseases, with their different aetiologies, can be divided rather crudely into two large groups:

1. Those with obvious genital symptoms: syphilis, gonorrhoea, chlamydial infection, chancroid and infections with some of the human herpesviruses (HHV1, HHV2 and HHV8), and in the long term, infection with some of the human papilloma viruses.
2. Those without obvious genital symptoms: infection with human immunodeficiency virus (HIV), hepatitis B virus (and perhaps with less certainty, hepatitis C virus), and some herpesviruses, especially HHV4.

In many infectious diseases the epidemiology is conditioned – among other factors – by the social environment of the population at risk. This includes the current moral climate. As an example, among the Fore people of New Guinea it was believed that eating the tribal elders when they died was an honourable and respectful thing to do. The brains were consumed especially by the women and children. It was they who suffered most heavily from Kuru, a spongiform encephalopathy with histological features similar to the reputedly new form of Creutzfeld–Jakob disease which, it has been suggested, may have been acquired by eating beef from animals with bovine spongiform encephalopathy. It took the force of law to change the climate of opinion among the Fore about 30 years ago, with the result that Kuru is no longer a problem, although sporadic cases still occur because of the occasional very long incubation period of this spongiform encephalopathy.

Sexually transmitted diseases are probably even more conditioned by the social environment than other infectious diseases, but it would certainly be more difficult to change the attitudes of the majority of humans to sexual activity than it was to alter the Fore mourning rituals. Although the official moral view in western societies is that unrestricted sex is a bad thing, the sexual behaviour of most humans seems to be incorrigible. Even when they know the risks, they still put themselves at hazard by exposing themselves to the possibility of infection. A fuller understanding of the epidemiology and pathology of sexually transmitted diseases may provide methods of limiting their spread by less drastic prescriptions than a demand for complete chastity.

## Syphilis

This worldwide infection is caused by the spirochaete *Treponema pallidum*. When it emerged in Europe at the end of the fifteenth and beginning of the sixteenth century its dissemination – especially in Italy, torn by a bitter and ferocious war between Spain and France – was promoted by civil disruption and the apparently unbridled licentiousness and brutality of the soldiery. To the French it was 'the Italian disease', to the Italians and Spaniards it was 'the French disease'. The tendency to blame the neighbours exists still. Five hundred years ago the infection was clearly far more virulent than it is today when the case fatality rate of untreated chronic syphilis may reach 30%. A high proportion of those infected in the fifteenth and sixteenth centuries died in the acute stages of the disease. This was perhaps because the virulence of the epidemic strain was exalted by rapid passage in a susceptible population (this is a well-known laboratory manoeuvre for selecting pathogenic strains of increased virulence in experimental situations), or simply because the affected population had little or no innate resistance to the treponeme; but the reason is now not known. It may be instructive to compare the evolution of syphilis in human populations with the evolution of myxomatosis in rabbits, discussed in Chapter 1.

The spirochaete passes readily from an infected woman to her fetus via the placenta. Until the development by Ehrlich in the years before the First World War of an effective treatment, congenital syphilis was a relatively frequent finding in infants in all classes of society. Before Ehrlich's Salvarsan was introduced in 1910 the majority of congenitally infected infants survived, but with a variety of deficits, though some later developed more serious and life-threatening manifestations of the disease.

The vast majority of *T. pallidum* infections are transmitted by the sexual route. The treponeme not only enters the new host through damaged skin, but is also able to penetrate undamaged mucous membranes. Spread from the infection site is rapid, both by the lymphatics and blood stream. Local treatment is thus useless. After an incubation period of, usually, 3 weeks the infected subject develops a lesion (the hard chancre) at the entry site of the organism. The chancre – a painless, indurated ulcer – is accompanied by a regional lymphadenopathy. Large numbers of treponemes can be seen by dark-ground microscopy of serous fluid from the chancre, and the lesion is extremely infectious. In heterosexual men the common sites of the primary lesion are the glans penis, the coronary sulcus and the inner aspect of the foreskin; although it may be found anywhere on the penis or adjacent parts. In the passive partner of a male homosexual relationship the chancre is most usually found in the anal canal, though it may be present in the mouth. In women, the chancre is found typically on the vulva, but it may be missed if it is on the cervix. The lesion heals within 2–6 weeks of it appearance.

Between 4 and 6 weeks later, the secondary stage of the disease becomes apparent. Many organs and systems are affected, but the visible form is of a symmetrical rash without itching or other irritation, and a generalized non-tender lymphadenopathy. The later the secondary rash develops, the larger the individual lesions are. Treponemes are present, making secondary syphilis contagiously infectious. Because the infection is so widely disseminated in the organs and systems of the body, symptoms may occur in relation to many of them. Clinical diagnosis of syphilis, except in the primary and the more typical secondary stages, is not easy. Because so many organs are involved the disease is a great mimic. When it was more common than it is today, it used to be said that to know syphilis was to know medicine. The secondary stage today is seldom as florid as it was even as relatively recently as the seventeenth and eighteenth centuries, when the size of the lesions caused the disease to be known as the great pox, to distinguish it from the smallpox. When the secondary stage clears up most subjects become non-infectious and the disease latent, but about a quarter may suffer infectious relapses during the next year or two. During the early part of latency pregnant women may infect their fetuses.

During the latent period infected persons may have no further symptoms for the rest of their lives, but in about 40% signs of destructive disease may appear in bone, mucous membranes and skin. Also large blood vessels – especially the aorta – and the central nervous system may be involved and lead eventually to the death of the patient. These stages, however, are of minimal epidemiological importance.

The most obvious control measure is to find and treat cases. This is most effectively done by tracing the contacts of patients diagnosed at special clinics. Syphilis is no longer the ubiquitous disease it was in the period before the introduction of effective treatment, and especially since the introduction of penicillin. About a fifth of new cases in England and Wales are in homosexual men. This segment of the population is also heavily involved in the transmission of syphilis in the USA (Wasserheit, 1994). Education in safe sex practices among homosexual men as part of the effort to reduce the incidence of infection with HIV should lead to reduction of syphilis too. Although syphilis is no longer a widely present health hazard in Britain, there is still a high incidence in parts of the developing world and in the USA. Over a period of 3 years, two-thirds of the new cases in a London STD clinic were infected by heterosexual contacts in foreign parts (Barlow and Sherrard, 1992).

In the USA the incidence of syphilis was reduced by almost 95% after the Second World War, but it later increased again, to reach 20 per 100 000 by 1990. Although the earlier part of the increase was mainly in homosexual men, between 1985 and 1990 the rate in heterosexual blacks increased by 165%, while decreasing among all other races. In 1985 the syphilis rate was 14 times greater in blacks than in whites; by 1991 the difference had increased to 60-fold (Gershman and Rolfs, 1991). This startling disparity may be related to the differences in socioeconomic circumstances between whites and the majority of the blacks in the USA.

The treatment of syphilis, as of all the classical or genitally apparent sexually transmitted diseases, should be conducted (or at the very least, supervised) by physicians who have special expertise in the field, as should the follow-up of each case for late complications and sequelae.

## Gonorrhoea

This disease, which was perhaps the most prevalent sexually transmitted disease in Britain, appears to be less pervasive than formerly. New cases occur predominantly in the younger age groups, with the highest incidence between ages 20 and 34; between 1981 and 1994 new cases in men decreased by 82%, and in women by 84% (Communicable Disease Report, 1996a). This decrease may have resulted from improved case finding and more successful treatment. It is unlikely to be the result of sexual intercourse protected by condoms, since the incidence of venereal chlamydial infection has, after a steep increase between 1981 and 1985, remained more or less stable with, latterly, a small decrease in females. In the USA the incidence of gonorrhoea has failed to decrease only in the age group 15–19 years. This is probably attributable to several factors, among which are the younger age of menarche in girls, and an increase in teenage sex, possibly encouraged by the general ambiance of society and the exploitation of sex in advertising, films, television and literature. The disease is caused by infection with the Gram-negative coccus *Neisseria gonorrhoeae*. The microorganism has no other host than human beings, and outside the body is highly vulnerable to atmospheric drying; but its direct transmission from person to person during sexual intercourse ensures that it seldom leaves the warm, moist environment in which it flourishes.

After a short incubation period – on average from 3 to 5 days – in men, the first sign is usually a discharge of pus from the urethra and discomfort on micturition. This develops into a more severe acute urethritis with continuing discharge of pus and a burning sensation on passing urine. About 5–10% of infected men have no symptoms and are thus liable to spread the infection without realizing it. Untreated, gonorrhoeal infection in men ends spontaneously, but several complications may occur. These are mainly local, such as abscess formation in any of the several groups of glands in various parts of the genitourinary system. A potentially serious late complication of untreated gonorrhoea – seen rather frequently in pre-antibiotic days – is stricture of the urethra, which may cause progressive urinary obstruction usually accompanied by urinary infection and the manifold associated problems

In women, the uterine cervix is the commonest site of infection, but both the urethra and the rectum may be involved. The incidence of symptomless infection in women is high – at least half not only have no symptoms, but examination reveals little or nothing to arouse suspicion. Correct diagnosis depends on bacteriological examination of samples of cervical mucus. Untreated or inadequately treated gonorrhoea is responsible for much preventable chronic disease. In women, gonorrhoea is a common cause of chronic pelvic inflammatory disease which is responsible for much infertility and ill health. With the proviso that the earlier treatment is instituted the better, adequate doses of penicillin rapidly cure those infections caused by sensitive strains of the gonococcus.

Diagnosis and treatment of sexually transmitted diseases is clearly important in controlling the spread of these infections. Bacteriological and serological investigation of all patients presenting at a clinic for STD should be regarded as obligatory. In addition to the isolation and identification of *N. gonorrhoeae*, tests for syphilis must always be made, since double infections are not unknown, and the treatment of gonorrhoea may mask the later occurring signs of syphilis and interfere with subsequent serological tests. Most strains of *N. gonorrhoeae* are still sensitive to penicillin; of those which are not, some produce an enzyme ($\beta$-lactamase) which actively destroys the antibiotic. Nevertheless, when the proper tests are made on strains isolated from patients, a suitable antibiotic can be selected and used for successful treatment. It is, however, important that the treatment should be supervised by a physician experienced in this branch of medicine.

To ensure that treatment has effectively removed a source of infection, cases should be followed up clinically and, where indicated, by laboratory investigation. Men with uncomplicated gonorrhoea should be told to return to the clinic if the treatment has not abolished the symptoms swiftly, or if they reappear. They should, in any case, be re-examined 1 week after treatment to ensure the absence of the complication of postgonococcal urethritis. In homosexual men gonococcal infection of the pharynx or the rectum is not uncommon. It is also more difficult to eradicate than urogenital gonorrhoea. Before a clean bill of health can be given, two negative cultures, a week apart, are required. Women, too, must return two successive weekly negative cultures to ensure the eradication of the infection. Since sexual activity seems to be less inhibited than formerly, women, too, may suffer pharyngeal and rectal in addition to cervical infection; all these sites should be investigated. All patients should be retested to exclude syphilis 2 months after the conclusion of the treatment.

As with syphilis, special care should be taken in case finding. The sexual partners of patients with gonorrhoea should be diligently sought, since some – especially women – may be free of symptoms despite being infected, and thus act as unknowing sources of infection in the community. It is not unusual to discover chains of infection which can be traced back to a particular infected person or group. The 1950s film *Carousel*, set in pre-first war Vienna, demonstrates entertainingly just how such a chain can be unwittingly established.

Babies born to infected mothers may be infected through

exposure to infected secretions in the birth canal. The routine instillation of a drop of dilute silver nitrate solution into each eye minutes after birth reduced the incidence of gonococcal ophthalmia neonatorum to virtually nil. This ophthalmia still occurs where there is a high incidence of gonorrhoea and inadequate health services, but in more developed regions such ophthalmia of the newborn as occurs is caused by other agents, especially *Chlamydia trachomatis*.

Not only syphilis and gonorrhoea, but all sexually transmitted infections, are likely to be more prevalent in social environments where overcrowding and poor hygiene are rife, and in situations where promiscuity is unrestrained, as among African truck drivers, whose routes appear to act as conduits of infection between towns and the rural areas they traverse (Bwayo *et al.*, 1991).

## Chlamydial infections

*Chlamydia trachomatis* and *C. psittaci* are the only species recognized in the genus *Chlamydia*. Both are widespread, and cause infections of humans, but only *C. trachomatis* appears to be a primary human pathogen. *C. psittaci*, first isolated in 1930, has been found in many different species of birds and mammals. Human infections are acquired, especially, from infected birds which are often symptomless. Occasional person-to-person transmission has been reported.

Chlamydiae are strict intracellular parasites. They are unable to synthesize ATP or high-energy phosphate bonds and are completely dependent on their host cells for all their energy needs; however because they synthesize their own DNA, RNA, and proteins they are clearly not viruses.

There are 15 major serotypes of *C. trachomatis*. A, B, and C occur in eye-to-eye transmission of trachoma, D to K in infections of male and female genital tracts, and L1, 2 and 3 in lymphogranuloma venereum (see below).

*C. trachomatis* is the causative agent of trachoma, a worldwide infection causing follicular conjunctivitis, responsible for much preventable blindness. The organism is spread either by direct transfer of secretions from an infected eye, or by indirect transfer of such secretions by flies. It is also transmissible by sexual intercourse, when it infects the urogenital tract and may cause acute or chronic infections in both men and women. Venereal infection of the conjunctiva with genital serotypes may occur. The infection of babies with genital serotypes during the birth process causes neonatal chlamydial ophthalmia, with an incubation period usually of 5–14 days. The infection can be aborted by topical application of tetracycline, erythromycin, or rifampicin eye ointment three times daily for 5 or 6 weeks, or erythromycin syrup by mouth for 3 weeks.

Between 1981 and 1995 genital infection with *C. trachomatis* increased approximately fourfold in women and twofold in men (Communicable Disease Report, 1996b). In 1995, 7226 cases were reported in men, and 17 536 in women. Sexually transmitted *C. trachomatis* is responsible in men for much non-gonococcal urethritis. The organism has been isolated from about 50% of men with gonococcal urethritis and 80% with postgonococcal urethritis. This association may be fortuitous, since both infections are likely to be found in the same type of patient – one who is promiscuous, not scrupulous in personal hygiene, and prone to repeated infections. Clinical suspicion of the diagnosis is confirmed by the isolation and identification of the organism. Treatment is usually effective. It is, however, important to treat the sexual partner(s) of these patients at the same time, to prevent reinfection, and in women to prevent acute non-gonococcal pelvic inflammatory disease.

In women attenders at clinics for STD, inflammation of the cervix is a common finding. *C. trachomatis* may be isolated from almost a third; but around two-thirds of women with gonorrhoea, or those whose sexual partners have non-gonococcal urethritis, also yield positive cultures. In women with adult chlamydial ophthalmitis, whose babies have the neonatal infection, the proportion with positive cultures is about 90%. Patients with cervical inflammation often develop pelvic inflammatory disease (PID). A third or more of patients with PID are infected with *C. trachomatis*. Treatment with tetracycline antibiotics must not be given to pregnant women because of their harmful effects on fetal bone and tooth development. Sexual partners of patients should be treated simultaneously, to prevent reinfection. Since a high proportion of infected women have no symptoms, their detection and treatment helps to reduce the reservoir of infection in the community.

Such a widespread infection seems an ideal subject for control by immunization. Several candidate vaccines have been investigated. None conferred more than very brief immunity but, in addition, made the recipients hypersensitive to chlamydial antigens.

Lymphogranuloma venereum is caused by *C. trachomatis* of serotypes L1, L2 and L3. The brunt of the infection is borne by lymphatic tissue. Although it is found in all parts of the world, the major centres of endemicity are in tropical and subtropical Africa, the Caribbean region, South America and South East Asia. Males and females are probably equally susceptible to infection, but the reported incidence in men is much greater than in women – perhaps because the early stages are more readily recognized in men. Infection is transmitted by both hetero- and homosexual intercourse. In the developed world the disease is most commonly diagnosed in travellers returning from endemic foci.

Clinical suspicion should be confirmed by laboratory investigation – either an immunofluorescence test or isolation in chick embryo yolk sac.

## Chancroid

This condition is caused by infection with *Haemophilus ducreyi* and is of minor importance in the developed world, except in the USA.

## Herpes simplex

This virus is an extremely common cause of venereal infection. Its two serotypes have different targets. Type 1 is reputed to infect above, and type 2 below, the belt – type 1 causing cold sores, etc., and type 2, venereal infections. This is, of course, not an absolute difference between the two, and since the sexual revolution of the 1960s and the more imaginative forms of sexual behaviour which accompanied it, the serotype of any isolate cannot be assumed from the site of the infection. Both types may be found in either situation, but venereal infections are still predominantly type 2. An outstanding feature of infection by all the known viruses of the herpes group is their ready assumption of latency. Herpes simplex virus becomes latent in the nervous system. Following buccal or pharyngeal infection it localizes in the Gasserian ganglion of the facial nerve, while the site of latency in venereal infections is the presacral ganglion.

Infectious sexual intercourse is followed by the appearance of lesions after an incubation period of 2–4 days. In both sexes the primary attack is accompanied by fever and malaise. In males the lesions – progressing from erythema to papules to vesicles – occur on the glans penis, the coronal sulcus and the shaft of the penis, and occasionally on the scrotum or the adjacent inner aspect of the thigh. Like the lesions of labial herpes they are irritating and painful, but after a few days they dry up and crust over, with subsequent separation of the scabs. In women the lesions may be difficult to see or, in the primary attack, be confined to the cervix. The attack is generally extremely painful and, as in men, preceded by prodromal sensations of itching and burning. Although dysuria may occur in both sexes it is more of a feature in women.

At some point in the course of the infection the virus enters one of the sacral nerves and is conveyed to the presacral ganglion where its DNA is integrated into the DNA of the infected ganglion cell. From time to time the virus is reactivated and distributed to the site (or close to it) of the primary infection, and there establishes a recurrent attack of genital herpes. Recurrent attacks are generally preceded by prodromal warnings similar to those experienced earlier. Clearly, the sufferer is highly infectious during an attack, but is not necessarily non-infectious as soon as the lesions heal. Some subjects of both sexes, but especially women with a cervical infection, may continue to excrete virus for many days. Early treatment of the primary attack with acyclovir may prevent latency, but this depends on very early, accurate diagnosis. The same drug may abort recurrent attacks if used soon enough after the appearance of prodromata, and may be expected to reduce the length of the attack and speed the healing. There is no vaccine. The only practicable prophylaxis is extreme care in choice of sexual partners and avoidance of unprotected intercourse.

The epidemiology of the group of sexually transmitted diseases with genital symptomatology is well understood, and treatment – for those where therapeutic agents exist – can be effective, particularly when applied by physicians specializing in this field of medicine. However, one of the aims of epidemiology is to indicate ways of preventing diseases – an aim which, in this group of infections, is woefully unmet. This is not to be ascribed to deficiencies in the epidemiological approach, but to the vagaries of human behaviour which conditions, and is conditioned by, the social environment in which people find themselves. This is well illustrated by the results of surveys made in 1990 and 1991 in Torbay, a seaside holiday resort area in Devon, England (Ford and Inman, 1992). More than 1500 people – locals, migrant holiday workers and holiday makers, between the ages of 16 and 29 – were interviewed. Almost one-third of them had sexual intercourse with at least one new partner while on holiday, but significantly fewer than half of these had used a condom. As a result, the Torbay public health department set up a wide-ranging 'sea, sand and safer sex' project for 1993. The effect of the project was assessed in the summer holiday season in 1994 by interviewing more than 300 young holiday makers in Torquay, the major Torbay holiday town. More than two-thirds of those who had attended project events, which combined entertainment with education, had read the leaflets available, talked with specially trained peer educators, and 'felt that the health messages were relevant to them'. Despite this the survey revealed considerable sexual networking, regular use of condoms by only 40%, and no use of any contraception by 17%.

In the absence of vaccines (except hepatitis B vaccine) against sexually transmitted diseases – the development of which seems improbable at present – 'old fashioned' case finding and treatment must continue to be relied upon as the main instrument in the control of these diseases, since education in safe practices – at least in Britain – is clearly not as effective as it should be.

## Hepatitis B

In parts of Africa, among Australian Aborigines, and in other parts of the world, the virus of hepatitis B may be transferred in blood on the instruments used during ritual ceremonies involving circumcision, tattooing, scarification, etc. It is also spread sexually – not only by prostitutes, who have a very high carrier rate, but also by male homosexuals who, in several parts of the world (notably New York and California) also have very high carrier rates. The customary sexual behaviour (which is not regarded locally as immoral) in much of Africa and among Australian Aborigines is a potent vehicle of transmission. The very high carrier rate in prostitutes and male homosexuals suggested the prime importance of the sexual route in the epidemiology of hepatitis B. However, the disease is also prevalent in closed societies such as orphanages and homes for the mentally subnormal where the sexual route ought to be of minor, if any, importance; but because of rather too frequent reports of hanky-panky in such establishments, transmission by routes other than sexual should not be accepted without close enquiry. There is no doubt, however, that hepatitis B virus may be transferred by mouth. There is also a considerable risk that mothers who are carriers may pass the infection to their infant children – especially if they have only recently become carriers – but the exact mechanism is not understood.

Surveys of serum samples for antibody to hepatitis B virus have revealed a vast number of carriers of the virus – about 200 000 000 worldwide. Most of this enormous reservoir is present in Africa, Asia and Latin America. It is probably more than a coincidence that these are the areas of the world with the greatest incidences of primary cancer of the liver. This is a rather rare neoplasm in the countries of the developed world, but in black Africans and in South East Asia it is among the most common cancers. This is not to say that hepatitis B virus is the sole cause of primary cancer of the liver, although there is a highly significant correlation between hepatocellular carcinoma and markers of infection by hepatitis B virus (Tswana and Moyo, 1992). There is little doubt that hepatitis B virus is an important part of a chain of factors involved in the aetiology of primary liver-cell cancer, one of which is aflatoxin produced by certain strains of the mould *Aspergillus niger* which thrives in warm, moist, tropical environments where storage facilities for foodstuffs are inadequate. In West Africa, ground nuts – important in the diet – are often contaminated. Thus the toxin has ready access to the cells and metabolic pathways of the liver. Whether accessory agents are needed for the virus to initiate the liver cancer is uncertain, but transgenic mice with a gene cloned from hepatitis B virus have developed the condition.

After hepatitis B virus was identified, the risks of transmitting it by blood transfusion were greatly reduced by measures such as selection of blood donors and testing of donated blood. The chance of infecting a patient via blood or blood products was excluded with a high degree of certainty. Nevertheless, cases of hepatitis clearly related to blood transfusion continued to occur, although at a reduced rate. The condition was labelled non-A non-B hepatitis.

## Hepatitis C

Most non-A non-B hepatitis is caused by hepatitis C virus. Persistent infection with the virus may occur in almost all who are infected, even in the absence of active liver disease (Alter *et al.*, 1992); but a high rate of chronic hepatitis and other liver diseases may be found many years after the original infection. There was a suspicion that hepatitis C virus, too, might be transmitted sexually, but the likelihood of this occurring seems to be small. An investigation of 170 heterosexual couples found 18% of the women and 33% of the men were positive for hepatitis C virus. Injecting drug use and a history of blood transfusion were both significantly associated with seropositivity for the virus, but the sexual behaviour of couples was not. However, two of 31 women with no history of parenteral risk who had long-term relationships with seropositive male partners were themselves seropositive, compared with none of 81 with seronegative male partners (Osmond, 1993). Phylogenetic trees of sequences of hepatitis C virus isolates from suspected heterosexual transmissions may be a useful method of determining the frequency of sexual transmission of the virus (Rice *et al.*, 1993; Holmes, 1996).

## Acquired Immune Deficiency Syndrome

This condition is generally known by its acronym, AIDS. The syndrome develops after a variable, but long, latent period after infection by the human immunodeficiency virus (HIV). Two serotypes of HIV are recognized. HIV-1 is overwhelmingly the more frequent virus found in Britain and most other parts of the world. Infections with HIV-2 are found predominantly in West Africa, but relatively recently HIV-2 infections have been found in India (Graz *et al.*, 1994), but at the time of writing had not moved far from the large towns and cities of the west coast (Lalvani and Shastri, 1996). The HIV-1 strains are of subtype C. This subtype and subtype E replicate very efficiently in Langerhans cells. Because these cells are found in genital mucous epithelia they may be the cells through which vaginal infection occurs in heterosexual spread of the virus. As in Africa, heterosexual spread is the predominant mode of transmission of HIV in India.

Although it has, retrospectively, been suggested that there was a death from AIDS in Manchester in 1959, phylogenetic analysis (Zhu and Ho, 1995) of virus isolated from preserved tissue threw doubt on the suggestion. The first recognized cases of AIDS were seen in San Francisco in 1980. They were linked with bizarre and rarely seen opportunistic infections such as pneumonia caused by the normally harmless protozoon *Pneumocystis carinii* (which was also present in the suspected Manchester case) and the appearance in young men of Kaposi's sarcoma, which is a rare tumour of older subjects in western societies. Other signs associated with the condition, such as lymphadenopathy and a dearth of lymphocytes, pointed to a massive failure of immunity; however, the cause was unknown. When it became apparent that similar involvement of the immune system was occurring in homosexual men in three centres in the USA, the cause of this newly recognized disease was ascribed to their general lifestyle, including the use of vasodilators such as glyceryl trinitrate to enhance sexual pleasure, before it was established that it was an infection, probably transmitted sexually.

The news that increasing numbers of homosexual men were being affected provoked more or less automatic statements by self-appointed moralists that the disease was a well-deserved punishment for their wicked behaviour, and no more than they deserved.

In the USA, which seems to be particularly beset by moralists of a kind which can best be described as Christian fundamentalists, it is widely believed that 'gay' white men have been singled out by this disease. This is not so, however: 'In the 96 largest metropolitan areas in the United States half all new HIV infections are transmitted through injecting drug use, a quarter through hetero-sexual intercourse (70–80% of these are in women), and only a quarter through homosexual intercourse …' (Merson, 1996). Despite the various routes and methods of transmission which have been described, in the world as a whole, more HIV is spread by heterosexual intercourse than by any other route. There are about 7500 new infections worldwide each day; half of them occur in Africa, where heterosexual intercourse is by far the most usual route. The origins of the viruses are unknown, but they may have been derived from a virus (or viruses) of African monkeys. Antibody to HIV has been demonstrated in samples of human serum collected in Africa and stored at sub-zero temperatures since the 1970s and earlier. The syndrome associated with infection by HIV almost certainly emerged quietly in Africa many years before it appeared so dramatically in the USA.

The virus is able to infect several different types of cell in the body of its host, the most important being lymphocytes expressing the CD4 molecule on their surfaces, i.e. helper T cells. It is also able to multiply in macrophages and other antigen presenting cells such as Langerhans cells. HIV can also infect certain cells in the brain, which leads, eventually, to dementia. When the virus enters the blood stream of a new host it attaches, with the aid of an accessory factor (or perhaps several accessory factors), to the surfaces of cells carrying the CD4 receptor, enters these cells, multiplies and – being a retrovirus – undergoes a complex process of integration in which the RNA genome is destroyed after being copied as the complementary DNA, and a second DNA chain is made, complementary to the first. The new DNA molecule is then integrated into the cellular genome. Some of the infected cells are killed and new HIV is set free to infect more $CD4^+$ cells, whose number is rapidly and severely reduced. The infected person may have a short illness with fever and lymphadenopathy, but recovers and is then well until the onset of the acquired immune deficiency syndrome (AIDS). During the latent period between the infection and the appearance of AIDS, which is variable, but may be long – sometimes as long as ten years – there is considerable production and turn-over of both virus and $CD4^+$ cells (Ho et al., 1995; Wei et al., 1995). When patients were treated with inhibitors of HIV proteases, the concentration of HIV-1 in the plasma decreased exponentially, with a mean half-life of about 2 days, while the numbers of CD4$^+$ lymphocytes increased considerably. These findings, which upset previously held views about the natural history of infection with HIV-1, should allow the establishment of a more hopeful therapeutic regimen for the infection, subject to the cost of the protease inhibiting drugs becoming affordable for the mass treatments that will be necessary. The constant, rapid turnover of virus allows it to be replaced frequently by mutant forms resistant to the immunity evoked by their forerunners, and, in the long run, promotes a steady depletion of the body's CD4$^+$ cells. This leads eventually to a reduction in the ability to respond positively to other infections, to such an extent that normally harmless microorganisms are able to establish opportunistic infections and disease. Patients infected with HIV remain infectious, however, no matter how healthy they appear. But it does seem that the virus load carried by the infected person during the latent period is more important than the number of immune cells in determining the timing of the outcome – which, as far as is known, is always fatal. Because of the rapid mutation of the virus, development of drug resistance is also rapid, although it is probable that treatment with several drugs simultaneously will not only be able to reduce the virus load for long periods, but will – it is hoped – also keep the emergence of resistance to a minimum.

The numbers of infected persons, both worldwide and in any particular country, are not known with certainty, but the World Health Organization (WHO) publishes estimates from time to time of the likely numbers of people with AIDS and those infected with HIV. The data suggest that by the end of 1994 there had been 4.5 million cases of AIDS worldwide since the onset of the pandemic (WHO, 1995). This is to be compared with just over a million cases reported to WHO by 31 December 1994. The discrepancy arises because of underdiagnosis, underreporting and delays in reporting. Of these, underreporting, which is probably the major contributor to the underestimating of cases, occurs because of policy decisions by many governments. Such decisions are made for a variety of reasons – economic, fear of losing tourist traffic, misplaced national pride and others – none of them creditable. The numbers infected with HIV, from which AIDS will in due course develop, are even more alarming. WHO estimates that at the end of 1994 there were between 13 and 15 million adults infected with the virus, more than half of them in subsaharan Africa. WHO also estimated that in some parts of the world – South and South East Asia, for example – the prevalence of infection with HIV is significantly greater (2.5 million adults) than even the reported number of AIDS cases (14 527) suggests. HIV infection is about 18% of all estimated infections, while AIDS cases reported to WHO in the South East Asia region are only 1.4% of all reported cases. It has been predicted that AIDS will be the leading cause of death in Thailand by the year 2000.

The incidence of infection with HIV, and its differential distribution in the population could be determined by stratified serological testing, but in the present climate of lay opinion, the knowledge that someone is infected with HIV may visit on him or her extremely adverse effects, both social and economic. It is, thus, clearly important to ensure the complete security of all results of seroepidemiological investigations. This has been achieved in England and Wales by the 'Unlinked Anonymous HIV Prevalence Monitoring Programme' in which, before testing residual samples of serum from routine clinical blood tests for the presence of markers of infection with HIV, they are stripped of all possibile identifying features of the patients concerned. The sera tested come from attenders at clinics for genitourinary medicine, i.e. homo- and bisexual men, and heterosexual men and women whose lifestyle and behaviour put them particularly at risk of infection with HIV (Gill et al., 1989). Samples are also tested from known injecting drug users. The results of the programme from its start in 1990 to 1993 have been published (Department of Health and Public Laboratory Service, 1993). The risk of infection in the population at large is estimated from the prevalence of maternal HIV infection. This is determined by testing the blood of newborn infants, whose antibody content reflects antibody transferred across the placenta, and is an indirect indicator of maternal infection. Blood samples are taken from infants by heel prick (Peckham et al., 1990).

It is clear from the Department of Health Report, as from other information, that high-risk behaviour, rather than a particular sexual orientation, is the main factor in determining the probability of acquiring HIV. In western societies the high-risk behaviour most likely to promote infection with HIV is unprotected penetrative anal intercourse between homosexual men. In the west, unprotected penetrative sexual intercourse between men and women is at present a less important, but increasing, high-risk behaviour, whereas in Africa and parts of South East Asia it is indubitably not only locally important, but also acts as a conduit for the transfer of infection from these reservoirs to those parts of the world where it is not yet a major factor in the circulation of the virus. HIV-1, subtype B, predominates in Europe and the Americas. Should subtype C (from Central and East Africa) gain a foothold in these geographical regions, it is likely that there will be a great increase in the heterosexual transmission of the virus because of the greater efficiency of the subtype's replication in the female genitalia.

In 1993 the greatest incidence of infection with HIV in England and Wales was in London and south-east England, and in this area the greatest prevalence was in homosexual and bisexual men between the ages of 25 and 44. The prevalence of infection in heterosexual men and women was low – less than 1%, except that in the age group 25–34 both men and women showed a prevalence of 1.3%. The Report from the Department of Health and Public Health Laboratory Service (1993) also presented evidence that, at least in two genitourinary clinics in central London, between 1990 and 1993 the prevalence of infection in homosexual men decreased from 22.3% to 17.3% – a statistically significant difference. Such a reduction does not necessarily indicate cessation of transmission, however, but can be accounted for by dead individuals being replaced by newly infected subjects at a reduced, but still measurable, rate. In any event, the high prevalence figures from these two clinics for infection in men younger than 25 suggests that their infections were probably recent, implying that too many in this age group are still engaging in high-risk practices. The continuing incidence of the traditional sexually transmitted diseases in this group confirms this view.

The prevalence of AIDS in heterosexual individuals in England and Wales (and probably in Britain as a whole) was still low in 1992, but had been – and still is – increasing more rapidly in individuals exposed heterosexually than in those exposed either homosexually or by sharing needles if injecting drug users (Communicable Disease Report, 1993).

Projections of prevalence rates depend on so many imponderables, especially judgements about future patterns of sexual behaviour, that close estimates of likely prevalences in the next several years are not really possible. Nevertheless, the increased prevalence of HIV infection in pregnant women in London, particularly in the age group 20–29 years, indicates the probability of heterosexual transmission of the virus becoming more common. Much of the heterosexually transmitted virus has an African origin: visitors to Africa have brought it back with them; visitors from Africa have brought it with them. In much of subsaharan Africa, where social conventions differ from those in the western world, and western ideas of sexual morality carry little weight, men and women engage in sexual intercourse very freely. An important consequence of this is that infection with HIV has reached serious epidemic proportions in many African countries, as shown by WHO's estimate of HIV prevalence quoted above. It is the fringes of this epidemic which have influenced, and are likely in future to continue influencing, the epidemiological situation in Britain, despite the suggestion (National Reports, 1994) that the incidence of AIDS may have reached a plateau in Germany, Switzerland and the UK.

Despite an immense investment in vaccine research since the importance of HIV infection was realized, until mid-1996 experimental vaccines were not particularly promising as potential candidate vaccines. Because the majority of infections with HIV occur during sexual intercourse, protective antibody should be present in adequate concentration at the point of exposure, i.e. the vaginal and rectal mucosae. This would require the presence on the threatened mucosal surface of secretory IgA of appropriate specificity. Lehner and colleagues (1996) subjected male rhesus monkeys to targeted immunization of the iliac lymph nodes with a recombinant vaccine of envelope and core polypeptides of simian immunodeficiency virus (SIV). Four of seven immunized animals were completely protected against rectal challenge with SIV and three were partially protected, i.e. had reduced viral load or a transient viraemia. Thirteen of the 14 control animals were infected by the challenge virus. The experimental route of immunization is clearly unsuitable for large-scale field or clinical use. However, protection against SIV having been demonstrated, the outlook for a prophylactic vaccine against the similar HIV is brighter than it has been; however, the waiting period for an acceptable vaccine will still be long.

Nevertheless, research on possible chemotherapeutic agents has, at the time of writing, begun to look more hopeful. Understanding of the complex biology and biochemistry of the virus replicative process has increased, allowing various compounds showing therapeutic activity to be synthesized which inhibit the action of HIV-specified proteases in infected cells. Such clinical trials as have been reported indicate rather strongly that even with compounds of high bioavailability there is a finite probability of resistant strains of virus arising; but this can be considerably reduced by combined treatment with several different protease inhibitors. Though not in any sense curative, such therapy, by appreciably reducing patients' virus loads, may be expected to prolong their useful lives.

Although the incidence of HIV infection and AIDS in Thai and African prostitutes is very high, there are indications that energetic encouragement of the use of condoms is having a positive effect in reducing the incidence of new HIV infections (Hanenberg et al., 1994; Lagu et al., 1994). Recently some of the African women – who have plied their trade for many years without the protection offered by condoms, which their customers generally refuse to use – were found to be apparently uninfected by HIV. When investigated they had increased concentrations of cytotoxic T lymphocytes (CD8$^+$ cells) (Langlade-Demoyen *et al.*, 1994; Rowland-Jones *et al.*, 1995). Some investigators have suggested that candidate HIV vaccines should be endowed with the ability to activate such CD8$^+$ cells as well as to stimulate antibody to selected surface epitopes of the virus. However, the transfer of HIV-1, *nef*-specific cytotoxic T lymphocytes to a patient with AIDS (Koenig *et al.*, 1995), was followed by a reduction in circulating CD4$^+$ cells and an increase in the patient's virus load. Virus isolated subsequently from the patient had lost the *nef* epitope. It was thus insensitive not only to the *nef*-specific cytotoxic cells, but also to any antibody specified by that epitope. Clearly, despite the encouraging report by Lehner *et al.* (1996), no easy or certain routes exist to an effective anti-HIV vaccine. HIV is, in any case, so genetically and antigenically labile that it is unlikely that any vaccine consisting of surface epitopes of the virus could have any long-term influence on the spread of the infection, since epidemic strains of the virus would simply mutate rapidly under the pressure of antibody stimulated by the vaccine strain(s), assuming that they were closely related to recently isolated field strains; if the vaccine had been derived from established laboratory strains of HIV the antibodies evoked would probably be of little, if any, significance.

In the longer term, it seems that control of the pandemic spread of HIV must depend more on changes in human attitudes to sexual gratification – which is to say, on changes in the social environment of both the sexually active and those censorious of virtually all sexual activity – than on a magic bullet produced by biomedical science. Probably the most important change would be a firm acceptance that, properly deployed, condom use is the next best preventive measure to total abstinence, and much more likely to be adopted, with proper encouragement from society at large. However, if the present, increasing, pandemic spread of the virus continues, mutational changes in both virus and humankind may be selected, which will lead, eventually, to the evolution of a situation like that between myxoma virus and Australian rabbits. But such an outcome must be many generations in the future, and is certainly not to be regarded as a sensible alternative to positive measures to stop people infecting each other.

# References

Alter, M.J., Margolis, H.S., Krawczynski, K. *et al.* (1992). The natural history of community-acquired hepatitis C in the United States. *New England Journal of Medicine* **327**, 1899–1905.

Barlow, D. and Sherrard, J. (1992). Heterosexual spread of HIV infection. *British Medical Journal* **305**, 179–180.

Bwayo, J.J., Omari, M.M., Mutere, A.N. *et al.* (1991). Long distance truck drivers: 1. Prevalence of sexually transmitted diseases (STDs). *East African Medical Journal* **68**, 425–429.

Communicable Disease Report (1993). AIDS and HIV-1 infection in the United Kingdom: monthly report. *Communicable Disease Report* **3**(4), 17.

Communicable Disease Report (1994). Infections and congenital syphilis in England. *Communicable Disease Report* **4**(20), 93.

Communicable Disease Report (1996a). Sexually transmitted diseases quarterly report: gonorrhoea in England and Wales. *Communicable Disease Report* **6**(13), 110–111.

Communicable Disease Report (1996b). Sexually transmitted diseases quarterly report: general infection with *Chlamydia trachomatis* in England and Wales. *Communicable Disease Report* **6**(22), 190–191.

Department of Health and Public Health Laboratory Service (1993). Unlinked Anonymous HIV Seroprevalence Monitoring Programme in England and Wales, data to the end of 1993.

Ford, N. and Inman, M. (1992). Safer sex in tourist resorts. *World Health Forum* **13**, 77–80.

Gershman, K.A. and Rolfs, R.T. (1991). Diverging gonorrhea and syphilis trends in the 1980s: are they real? *American Journal of Public Health* **81**, 1263–1267.

Gill, O.N., Adler, M.W. and Day, N.E. (1989). Monitoring the prevalence of HIV. Foundation for a programme of unlinked anonymous testing in England and Wales. *British Medical Journal* **299**, 1295–1298.

Graz, M., Dietrich, V., Balfe, P. *et al.* (1994). Genetic analysis of HIV-1 and HIV-2 mixed infections in India reveals a recent spread of HIV-1 and HIV-2 from a single ancestor for each of these viruses. *Journal of Virology* **68**, 2161–2168.

Hanenberg, R.C., Rojananpithaykorn, W., Kunasol, P. and Sokal, D. (1994). Impact of Thailand's HIV-control programme as indicated by the decline in sexually transmitted diseases. *Lancet* **344**, 243–245.

Ho, D.D., Neumann, A.U., Perelman, A.S. *et al.* (1995). Rapid turnover of plasma virions and CD4 cells in HIV-1 infection. *Nature* **373**, 123–126.

Holmes, E.C. (1996). Reconstructing the history of viral epidemics. *Biologist* **43**, 54–57.

Koenig, S., Conley, A.J., Brewah, Y.A. *et al.* (1995). Transfer of HIV-1-specific cytotoxic T lymphocytes to an AIDS patient leads to selection for mutant HIV variants and subsequent disease progression. *Nature Medicine* **1**, 330–336.

Lagu, M., Alary, M., Nzila, N. *et al.* (1994). Condom promotion, sexually transmitted disease, treatment, and declining incidence of HIV-1 infection in female Zairian sex workers. *Lancet* **344**, 246–248.

Lalvani, A. and Shastri, J. S. (1996). HIV epidemic in India: opportunity to learn from the past. *Lancet* **347**, 1349–1350.

Langlade-Demoyen, P., Ngo-Glang-Huong, N., Ferchal, F. and Oskenhendler, E. (1994). HIV nef-specific cytotoxic T lympohocytes in noninfected heterosexual contacts of HIV-infected patients. *Journal of Clinical Investigation* **93**, 1293–1297.

Lehner, T., Wang, Y., Cranage, M. *et al.* (1996). Protective mucosal immunity elicited by targeted iliac lymph node immunization with a subunit SIV envelope and core vaccine in macaques. *Nature Medicine* **2**, 767–775.

Merson, M.H. (1996). Returning home: reflections on the USA's response to the HIV/AIDS epidemic. *Lancet* **347**, 1673–1676.

National Reports to the European Centre for the Epidemiological Monitoring of AIDS (1994). *AIDS Surveillance in Europe.* Quarterly Report No. 44, 31 December.

Osmond, D.H., Padian, N.S., Sheppard, H.W. *et al.* (1993). Risk factors for hepatitis C virus seropositivity in heterosexual couples. *Journal of the American Medical Association* **269**, 361–365.

Peckham, C.S., Tedder, R.S., Biggs, M. *et al.* (1990). Prevalence of maternal HIV infection based on unlinked anonymous testing of newborn babies. *Lancet* **335**, 516–519.

Rice, P.S., Simmonds, P., Smith, D.B. and Holmes, E.C. (1993). Heterosexual transmission of hepatitis C virus. *Lancet* **342**, 1052–1053.

Rowland-Jones, S., Sutton, J., Ariyoshi, K. *et al.* (1995). HIV-specific cytotoxic T-cells in HIV-exposed but uninfected Gambian women. *Nature Medicine* **1**, 59–64.

Tswana, S.A. and Moyo, S.R. (1992). The interrelationship between HBV-markers and HIV antibodies in patients with hepatocellular carcinoma. *Journal of Medical Virology* **37**, 161–164.

Wasserheit, J.N. (1994). Effects of changes in human ecology and behavior on patterns of sexually transmitted diseases, including human immunodeficiency virus infection. *Proceedings of the National Academy of Science of the USA* **91**, 2430–2435.

Wei, X., Ghosh, S.K., Taylor, M.E. *et al.* (1995). Viral dynamics in human immunodeficiency virus type 1 infection. *Nature* **373**, 117–122.

WHO (1995). WHO AIDS data at 31 December 1994 and the current global situation of the HIV/AIDS pandemic. *Weekly Epidemiological Record* **70**, 5–8.

Zhu, T. and Ho, D.D. (1995). Was HIV present in 1959? *Nature* **374**, 503–504.

# Chapter 7

# Some gastrointestinal infections

The gastrointestinal tract is subject to invasion by a wide range of organisms: various worms, protozoa, yeasts, bacteria and viruses. Although all of these types of organisms may cause diseases, either life threatening or chronically debilitating, infections by bacteria and viruses are probably responsible for more serious morbidity than any other group. The infections to be discussed in this chapter are cholera (at some length), bacterial food poisoning caused by *Bacillus cereus,* enterotoxinogenic *Staphylococcus aureus, Salmonella* spp., and *Campylobacter* spp., and infection by rotavirus and some other viruses. As noted above, these are not the only infectious causes of intestinal disease, but they are important, not only numerically, but also because they illustrate so clearly the relationship between infection and environment.

## Cholera

A study of the distribution of a disease may give clues to its causation. A single example shows this very clearly. Cholera was endemic in London from about 1830. During an epidemic outbreak, John Snow, a physician living in Soho, was struck by the different incidences of the disease in different parts of the quarter. In the vicinity of the pump at Broad Street (now named Broadwick Street), from which many households drew their water, the incidence was particularly high; but in the nearby workhouse there were only five cases among the 535 inhabitants. The workhouse drew water from its own well. Among the 70 men working in the Broad Street brewery there were no cases. The brewery had its own deep well, but the men drank little or nothing from it directly, preferring the beer which they brewed. From such data, and others on the incidence of cholera in the vicinity of other public water pumps in Soho, Snow constructed a map which showed clearly that the majority of cases were related to the Broad Street pump. In a famous gesture he sent his manservant to remove the pump handle. People had to use other pumps dispensing water supplied by a different company, and the outbreak of cholera, which was, in any case, beginning to wane, soon died away.

Snow later expanded his research by investigating the incidence of cholera in Soho households supplied with piped water by different water companies. The water delivered to many houses with high incidences of cholera among their inhabitants, like the water of the Broad Street pump, came from a part of the River Thames just below a raw-sewage outfall, while the water delivered by a different water company to other houses and pumps was much less polluted by sewage and also much less associated with cases of cholera. Snow concluded that there was something in the polluted water which caused cholera, but the *Vibrio cholerae* bacterium was not isolated until 1883, almost 30 years later, when Robert Koch showed it to be the responsible infectious agent.

The habitat of the causative organism, *Vibrio cholerae*, is saline water, in which it can survive and multiply in a range of salt concentrations. It is extremely sensitive to acid environments, but grows well in alkaline peptone water. Because of its lability at acid pH, the infecting dose in persons with normal gastric physiology is extremely large. In healthy, fasting adults, $10^9$ microorganisms do not regularly cause disease; but after a dose of antacid, or a meal containing much protein which neutralizes gastric acidity, infection may be produced by as few as $10^6$ bacteria. In endemic or epidemic situations people with achlorhydria, however caused, are at increased risk of infection. Those bacteria which pass through the stomach into the small bowel attach to the brush border of the intestinal mucosa and secrete the toxin which is responsible for the symptoms of the disease.

*Vibrio cholerae* may be found in water or food, especially fresh vegetables contaminated by the faeces of carriers or those suffering from the disease. Carriers with mild, or even no, symptoms may be involved in spreading epidemic cholera: only about 2% of people demonstrably infected with the El Tor biotype of the bacterium actually show signs of disease, although the bacteria which they excrete are infectious. Contaminated shellfish, especially bivalves, are potent sources of infection. The bacteria are either ingested and concentrated by the shellfish, or they multiply within the creatures. In either event, the flesh of the shellfish may contain very large numbers of microorganisms.

Until recently two variants of *Vibrio cholerae* were recognized, both of which carry the lipopolysaccharide surface antigen O1, and both of which occur in one or other of three serotypes, Ogawa,

Inaba and Hikojima. The variants are distinguishable by their *biotype* – the way they behave in culture. The classical biotype is sensitive to the antibiotic polymixin B and to group IV cholera bacteriophage, whereas the variant known as El Tor (named for the El Tor quarantine station in Sinai, where the first isolations were made as long ago as 1905) is not; and only the El Tor biotype is able to agglutinate fowl, sheep and human red blood cells. El Tor strains isolated up to 1962 were haemolytic, but more recent isolates have lost this activity. Because El Tor strains behaved differently in culture from classical cholera strains, received opinion in the 1930s, and even much later, held that the disease they caused was not cholera, but some other (indistinguishable) enteric inflammation. Understanding of the role of cholera toxin – secreted by all the pathogenic strains – in the pathogenesis of the disease has clarified the situation.

In October 1992 a third variant, carrying the antigen O139, was identified in Madras. It has caused epidemic outbreaks of disease indistinguishable from typical cholera in both India and Bangladesh (Cholera Working Group, 1993). It has also been isolated in Thailand. Infection with this strain does not confer protection against infection with strains carrying the O1 antigen. Since the enterotoxin secreted by O139 strains appears to be identical with that of the O1 strains, this suggests rather strongly that antitoxic immunity offers little, if any, protection against infection. In regions endemic for cholera, the brunt of any epidemic outbreak is borne by the children; although in newly invaded areas, and apparently in any area invaded by the new serotype O139, the incidence of infection and disease is more uniform in all age groups.

Since 1817, cholera has broken out from the Ganges delta and spread worldwide in seven pandemics. The seventh pandemic started in 1964 in Sulawesi (Indonesia). During the course of this pandemic, the El Tor biotype – first isolated in 1905 – almost completely replaced the classical biotype. The El Tor biotype was also responsible for an epidemic outbreak of cholera in the Celebes (Sulawesi) in 1937; however this was deemed at the time not to be true cholera, but a different intestinal inflammation with a virtually identical clinical picture. Some workers active in the cholera field believe that disease caused by infection with the O139 variant heralds the start of the eighth pandemic (Swerdlow and Ries, 1993). However, like El Tor strains, the new strains are able to agglutinate fowl erythrocytes (Cholera Working Group, 1993), and it has been suggested that it is not a non-O1 strain which has acquired toxinogenicity, but an antigenically mutated El Tor strain. The fact that isolates from sources as distant as Madras and Bangladesh have been shown by DNA probes to be clonal in origin strengthens this view. Outbreaks which it causes are more likely to be continuations of the seventh pandemic than the beginning of the eighth.

As recently as 1982 a firm statement was made that 'Under natural conditions, cholera vibrios produce attacks of diarrhoea, inapparent cases, and carrier states in no other animals than man' (Chatterjee, 1982). The inference to be drawn from this is that only man is infected by the organism. But *V. cholerae* had been isolated a few years earlier from the gut contents of intestinal worms excreted in the rice-water stools of cholera patients (Nalin and McLaughlin, 1977). The bacteria were – not surprisingly – present on the cuticle and mouth parts of the worms, but when worms (mainly mature females) were washed in acid to destroy adventitious vibrios before being sampled for culture, 28/32 had, in their intestines, *V. cholerae* of the same serotype that the patients had in their stools.

Many of the recent ecological studies of vibrios, and especially *V. cholerae* (Epstein, 1992; Epstein *et al.*, 1993), have shown that both phyto- and zooplankton act, at the least, as conveyors of *V. cholerae* for very long distances via ocean currents. Not only have non-culturable forms of *V. cholerae* been found in drinking water (Byrd *et al.*, 1991), but also such forms, with their greatly reduced metabolic rates, are able to survive by tolerating altered temperature, pH, salinity, and nutrient concentrations. Conditions conducive to algal blooms – increased nitrogen and phosphate in warmer water – allow the bacteria to revert to a culturable and infectious state. The key association is that with zooplankton: as many as $10^6$ bacteria have been found on copepod egg sacs; *V. cholerae* has also been found in the flesh of molluscs and in fish skin and intestines.

The warming of the sea may, in part, be a function of general global warming, although this cannot, yet, be accurately quantified. Another, demonstrable, cause of oceanic warming is the El Niño component of the Southern Oscillation – a combined meteorological and oceanographic phenomenon of great power and considerable influence on climatic conditions in many parts of the world (Philander, 1990). El Niño is the name given to the climatic change, originally along the west coast of South America, caused by the alteration in the direction of the wind and the increase in surface temperature of the sea which occurs from time to time in the tropical Pacific Ocean around Christmas. The name is a metaphor for the Christ Child, given to it by Peruvian fishermen many years ago, before its worldwide significance was understood. El Niño has a profound effect on climate and weather patterns – not just confined to the Pacific Ocean and the countries bordering upon it, but influencing Atlantic, European, African and Asian weather too. As long-term changes in the tilt of the earth increase the summer insolation of the southern hemisphere, and hence the surface temperature of the sea, the eastward current of warm water in the tropical Pacific Ocean so closely associated with the appearance of El Niño may be expected to occur more frequently; this, indeed, appears to be happening. Philander (1990) draws attention to the fact that: 'El Niño is now associated primarily with ecological and economic disasters that coincide with devastating droughts over the western tropical Pacific, and unusual weather patterns over various parts of the world'.

El Niño was present in 1990–91, 1992–93 and subsequently. In 1991 cholera appeared on the coast of Peru – probably carried in the ballast water of a ship from South East Asia, possibly as a passenger, in non-culturable form, on zooplankton – and spread rapidly along the Peruvian coast, presumably by the sea route, along virtually the whole of the west coast of South America, and via rivers, to Brazil, Venezuela and Bolivia. The prevention and control of epidemic outbreaks of cholera might seem to be difficult almost to the point of impossibility in the face of such rapid and widespread dispersion. However, prevention does not necessarily depend on the complete elimination of the pathogenic agent (although eradication does).

Dr John Snow showed in London about 150 years ago that the most important factor in controlling outbreaks of cholera is a clean water supply; such a supply can generally be relied upon to prevent outbreaks of water-borne cholera. However, the regions where cholera occurs most frequently are tropical and too poor to be able to afford the cost of modern water-treatment plants and supply reticulations. Their inhabitants' needs mean they must use river and pond waters, often heavily polluted by faeces. Infants suffer the greatest incidence, not only of cholera, but of other diarrhoeal diseases. In slum areas of the Third World the first 2 years of life are extremely hazardous for young children who suffer, on average, up to ten attacks of diarrhoeal disease in a single year, and as many as a third of deaths in children under 2 years of age result from dehydration and other complications of diarrhoea. The incidence of infection by *V. cholerae* and other intestinal pathogens diminishes with increasing age, while immunity increases. Deep wells with lined walls (tube wells) offer an improved water quality, where it is possible to install them. However, the long-term, permanent control of epidemic cholera is less of a medical problem than a problem of economics and engineering.

Current, commercially prepared, vaccines are not particularly effective, the better ones offering to adults 60–80% protection for 3–6 months – clearly inadequate for outbreak prevention and community protection. Even at the personal level, travellers are well advised to rely more on food and drink hygiene to prevent infection than to put their trust in vaccines. At present, therefore, epidemiological control of cholera by immunization is not a sensible option. In the medium term, however, there is the possibility of a rationally designed, live, oral anticholera vaccine being available (Suharyono *et al.*, 1992; Levine and Kaper, 1993). Such a vaccine has, at the time of writing, been licensed for use in Switzerland. There are sound reasons, both theoretical and experimental, for believing that properly engineered oral bacterial vaccines will confer better immunity, by stimulating the production of secretory IgA against intestinal infections, than the commonly available killed vaccines administered parenterally. Should oral vaccines be safe and effective in the field, as seems likely (Levine and Kaper, 1993) – and available at a price the poorest countries can afford – they would offer a more immediate opportunity to keep cholera within bounds until permanent public-health engineering developments make them no longer necessary. Since there is no possibility of eliminating choleragenic bacteria from the world, countries without piped supplies of adequately treated and monitored water will remain at risk of epidemic outbreaks of cholera should their immunization programmes with modern vaccines falter or break down.

## Bacterial food poisoning

Among the more important microorganisms associated with bacterial food poisoning are *Bacillus cereus, Campylobacter jejuni, Clostridium perfringens, Salmonella* spp., *Staphylococcus aureus, Vibrio parahaemolyticus* and *Yersinia enterocolitica*. All cause gastroenteritis which is generally self limiting, but may be life threatening in the very young, the debilitated and the old. Some are more important numerically than others. *Cl. perfringens, V. parahaemolyticus* and *Y. enterocolitica*, although very different kinds of microorganisms, probably share the attribute of being intrinsic in the milk or animal flesh (fish and shellfish, in the case of the vibrio) from which humans acquire their infection. Indirect person-to-person infection can, and does, occur when a carrier – usually either a domestic or a commercial food handler –

contaminates food which is subsequently eaten by family members, or members of the public at some sort of gathering such as a celebration. But carriers must acquire their infection somehow, and this may be by eating food containing something already contaminated before the preparation or processing began.

### *Bacillus cereus* food poisoning

*Bacillus cereus*, a Gram-positive spore-forming aerobe, is responsible for two types of food poisoning. In the *diarrhoeal syndrome*, the patient, after an incubation period of 8–16 hours, develops a profuse watery diarrhoea, often with anal tenesmus and sometimes with nausea and vomiting. Many different foods have been implicated: cooked meats and poultry, cooked vegetables, soups and sauces. The cooking process is not hot enough to destroy all spores in the food. The survivors germinate, multiply in the highly nutritious environment surrounding them, and produce their toxin. *B. cereus* is present in soils, hence vegetables (and, for some reason, especially spices) may be heavily contaminated. The diarrhoeal syndrome may thus be found particularly among people who use spices freely in their cuisine. Individual attacks last for 12–24 hours. The second manifestation, the *emetic syndrome*, occurring after an incubation period of 1–5 hours, is characterized by nausea, vomiting, and abdominal cramps, with diarrhoea occasionally, later. In Britain it is particularly associated with cooked rice which has been kept (especially by 'take-away' food retailers) from one day to the next without refrigeration. As the rice cools, spores which have survived the cooking process germinate and multiply (Gilbert *et al.*, 1974). Toxin is released during the logarithmic phase of growth of the microbes. Prevention of the condition is promoted by avoiding the practice of keeping unused cooked rice for another day.

### Staphylococcal food poisoning

Staphylococcal food poisoning follows the ingestion of food contaminated by an enterotoxin-producing strain of *Staphylococcus aureus*. Five different enterotoxins (A–E) have been identified, of which enterotoxin A is found most commonly. The staphylococci are able to multiply freely in many foods, and the toxin they secrete causes nausea, vomiting, abdominal pain and diarrhoea between 1 and 6 hours after the contaminated food has been eaten. A common source of the contamination is a food handler with an infected wound in a situation making the transfer of an inoculum of cocci a likely phenomenon. The contaminated food – mayonnaise, chicken salads, cream-based desserts, ice cream mix which is allowed to stand for long periods before being frozen, and similar items – becomes a vehicle for staphylococcal enterotoxin when it is left in a warm kitchen instead of being stored at a temperature of less than 5°C until it is needed for further processing, or until it is to be consumed.

The investigation of outbreaks of food poisoning includes not only the collection of clinical and historical data from patients and kitchen staff, but also the laboratory examination of clinical specimens from these people. Samples of suspect food should also be examined in the laboratory.

In all instances of bacterial food poisoning environment plays an important part. In staphylococcal food poisoning the relevant environment is that of the kitchen, which should be studied closely to determine at what stage(s) of preparation there are deficiencies in hygiene. Kitchen staff should be interviewed to assess their understanding of the importance of personal hygiene (including the prompt reporting of all wounds of the hands, and infections of other parts of the body), general kitchen cleanliness, and the prime necessity of refrigerating prepared foods if they are not to be consumed immediately.

### Salmonella food poisoning

With a few exceptions, such as *Salmonella typhi*, the paratyphi organisms and *Salmonella cholerae-suis* which cause systemic diseases, the vast majority of salmonella infections are confined to the gut where they cause severe, but usually self limiting, gastroenteritis – the diarrhoea and vomiting of bacterial food poisoning. Spread from person to person by the faecal–oral route is not only possible, but occurs all too frequently because of poor or non-existent personal and kitchen hygiene on the part of both domestic and commercial food handlers. However, since virtually all food-poisoning salmonellas make their initial entry into the human population via foodstuffs of animal origin, salmonella gastroenteritis must be regarded as a zoonosis; however, naturally occurring infection with *S. typhi* and the three paratyphoid salmonellas has no known animal source.

In England and Wales in 1994 there were almost 50 000 notifications of food poisoning to the Office of National Statistics. Not all of these were salmonella food poisoning, but about 30 000 salmonella infections in humans were reported in 1993 and a similar number in 1994 (Communicable Disease Report, 1994). Bacterial food poisonings of all kinds are almost certainly heavily under-reported, so the figures given are but a dim reflection of the real prevalence of food poisoning in general.

The ever-increasing number of food-poisoning salmonellas isolated from animal, human, and sometimes vegetable, sources are dignified by specific epithets – usually derived from their provenances – to distinguish them from each other. This makes them easier to talk and write about, but it should be remembered that the concept of species in bacteria is different from that in eukaryotic organisms. Salmonellas may be sorted into groups which are distinguished from each other by their somatic (O) antigens. Salmonella 'species' are largely determined by differences in serotype, determined by their flagellar (H) antigens, within a very large set of similar microorganisms. The three salmonellas occurring most commonly in human infections in Britain are *S. enteritidis, S. typhimurium,* and *S. virchow.*

Because of the industrialization of food production – especially the production of poultry – the dissemination of food-poisoning microorganisms has been greatly facilitated. The enormous number of birds – often many thousands – crowded into poultry sheds, provides a model environment for the rapid spread of pathogens. Infection of a very high proportion of the birds in a shed is a virtual certainty. *S. enteritidis* is the salmonella most usually associated with poultry, and various phage and serotypes of this microbe have largely supplanted *S. typhimurium* as the organism most commonly involved in outbreaks of salmonella food poisoning. Because so many chicken carcasses are infected, the further spread of salmonellas to uncontaminated carcasses is virtually unavoidable in the conditions under which these materials are handled in processing plants. Even in plants kept scrupulously clean, contamination of the water used for washing fowl carcasses can scarcely be prevented, so the salmonellas carried by infected birds are readily spread to most of the birds being processed.

The butchering of the carcasses of other meat animals is also, inevitably, associated with the mechanical spread of potentially pathogenic microbes. The contamination, derived from gut contents, is largely of the surfaces of the meats, which may, therefore, be consumed safely if simple hygienic measures are in use. A well-organized kitchen is needed where the risk of contamination of prepared foods by contact (direct or indirect) with raw, contaminated meats is prevented. Poultry and other meats should be cooked at temperatures, and for times, that will destroy the contaminating bacteria; and frozen meats and especially poultry should be completely thawed before being cooked. The advice given by the Department of Health about the use of eggs (Department of Health, 1988) should be adhered to, because of the high incidence of salmonella infection in poultry flocks and the ease with which it spreads.

Most domestic outbreaks of salmonella food poisoning result from failures of elementary hygiene, often because of ignorance. Outbreaks caused by commercially prepared foods (as at public receptions, weddings, etc.) generally result from carelessness, inadequate supervision of workers, failure to refrigerate prepared foods at sufficiently low temperatures, and generally ignoring advice about food hygiene which is offered liberally by health authorities.

It is scarcely an exaggeration to say that we are surrounded by epidemic bacterial food poisoning. It can also be said that salmonella food poisoning, like that caused by enterotoxinogenic staphylococci, can be ascribed to a widespread ignorance (and sometimes disregard) of the overwhelming importance of the environments, both physical and intellectual, in which food animals are produced and slaughtered, and foods are prepared.

### Campylobacter food poisoning

Campylobacter food poisoning is responsible for more bacterial food poisoning in Britain than any other microorganism (Pearson and Healing, 1992), including the salmonellas. In 1995 (Communicable Disease Report, 1996), for example, the total of food-poisoning cases reported to or otherwise ascertained by the Office of National Statistics was 83 346, while the number of confirmed cases of *Campylobacter* infection was 43 912 – more than half of all types of food poisoning.

Members of the genus have been recognized for more than 80 years as causing infectious abortion of cattle and sheep, when they were classified in the genus *Vibrio*. The genus *Campylobacter* was defined in 1963 (Sebald and Véron, 1963). The organisms are fastidious in their culture requirements and it was only in the second half of the 1970s that, with improved methods of isolation from faeces and other material, their importance as a cause of human disease became clear, and a scheme of classification was instituted.

Most *Campylobacter* disease is caused by *C. jejuni* and *C. coli*, but other species have, from time to time, been isolated from human clinical samples. The disease has an incubation period of between 2 and 10 days, and generally presents as a very copious watery diarrhoea with severe abdominal pain, and sometimes fever. It has been said that it can be distinguished from salmonella food poisoning in which the patient feels as though the bottom has dropped out of his world, while in campylobacter infection it is as though the world has dropped out of his bottom. Like other forms of bacterial food poisoning it is usually self limiting. It lasts for about a week to 10 days, though in some severely ill patients the condition may continue for as long as a month. The clinical diagnosis should be confirmed by isolation of the organism from faeces. Because this is not always attempted the condition tends to be underreported. A few patients – almost always old or debilitated – may die, but until the true incidence of infection is known no precise estimate can be made of the case fatality rate. Because it has had much less impact on the media than salmonella food poisoning, there has been correspondingly less reaction to it from the public.

*Campylobacter jejuni* has been found in the gut contents of many species, poultry, cattle, sheep, dogs, various wild animals and birds; and *C. coli* in the gut contents of pigs and poultry. These organisms are also found on the surface of many of the meats which are commonly in the diet, especially chicken. The numerous potential sources of infection leave no doubt that it is a major cause of diarrhoeal disease in persons of all ages in all parts of the world. Poultry, water and unpasteurized milk have clearly been shown to be the vehicle in several outbreaks of campylobacter disease, and must be regarded as major sources of human infections. Milk is presumably contaminated after it has left the cow – possibly by the entry of cow faeces. The microbes are destroyed by pasteurization, but in several outbreaks in 1990 and 1991 which were traced to bottled pasteurized milk, jackdaws and magpies were found to be pecking through the aluminium caps of milk bottles left on doorsteps and seeding the organisms in the contents (Hudson *et al.*, 1991). Campylobacters, as well as being found in a variety of animals, are also environmental organisms which have been isolated from rivers, lakes and the sea in many countries, including Britain. Water is presumably the source of infection for fish and shellfish, both of which may be responsible for human disease. The numbers of organisms recoverable from various waters may differ widely at different times of the year and, like vibrios, campylobacters can survive as viable but non-culturable entities (Rollins and Colwell, 1986).

Much of the domestic infection which occurs is most probably the result of unhygienic practices in the kitchen, stemming from ignorance and carelessness. Frozen poultry should be completely thawed before being adequately cooked, and chopping boards, work tops, and knives and other utensils should be carefully cleaned when the preparation of the food has been completed, to prevent the cross-contamination of cooked foods with potentially infective material from raw meats.

### *Helicobacter pylori* infection

This microorganism looks very like *Campylobacter jejuni* and is fairly closely related. It is present in high frequency in human duodenal and gastric ulcers. It is now reasonably certain that it is not merely a contaminant of the injured part of the intestinal mucous membrane, but plays a causal role in the pathogenesis of peptic ulcers. Successful treatment of the infection speeds the healing of the ulcer. A plausible mechanism has been proposed which explains how *H. pylori* stimulates the production of the excess gastric acid which is necessary for the development of ulcers. Successful treatment of the infection reduces acid production to normal and allows the damaged mucosa to regenerate and the ulcer to heal. Continued absence of the microorganism seems virtually to ensure that the ulcer does not recur.

*H. pylori* may be implicated in the development of gastric cancer. If so, about 60% of these cancers could be prevented by adequate treatment of the bacteria in the stomach. This is at present hypothetical, but some clinical findings suggest that the bacterium may be active in at least some stomach cancers. It is not clear how *H. pylori* gains access to the stomach and duodenum, but it has been found in dental plaque which may, therefore, act as a reservoir.

## Intestinal infection by viruses

Members of the enterovirus group and other viruses which infect the gut are widely disseminated throughout the world and with bacterial and other agents cause many millions of cases of diarrhoea annually, of which a high proportion end in death from dehydration. The brunt of these attacks falls on infants in the first 2 years of life. A very high proportion of the virus infections is caused by rotaviruses, which may be either food- or water-borne. More than 90% of rotavirus attacks occur in children less than 5 years old. The greatest morbidity and mortality are in those younger than 2. Since 80–100% of adults have circulating antibody against rotavirus, babies should be born with passive immunity to the virus; but if the antibody is not secretory IgA it will have little if any effect on virus within the lumen of the gut. Much – but clearly not all – of this disease and death would probably be avoided if mothers were not seduced by food-processing and pharmaceutical firms into substituting artificial baby-food formulas for breast feeding. Be that as it may, probably more infant gastrointestinal pathology results from infection with rotavirus than from any other cause.

Rotaviruses, which resemble little spoked wheels when viewed in the electron microscope, are associated with diarrhoeal disease in neonatal or young mammals of many species. Because rotaviruses are reluctant to grow in cell cultures, laboratory diagnosis depends on displaying the typical virus morphology by electron microscopy of samples of suspect stools. In Britain and other temperate-climate regions the incidence is largely seasonal, often increasing in early spring. In hot climates seasonality is not a feature; although this may have less to do with climate than the fact that most of the poorest countries with a high proportion of unhygienic living environments are in hot-climate regions.

Immunization against rotavirus infection would probably save many young lives. A conventional vaccine is excluded because of the difficulty of growing enough virus in cell cultures. A genetically engineered vaccine would be more likely; but because the greatest incidence of disease and death is in poor countries unable to afford the finished product, commercial interest in the manufacture of such a vaccine is likely to be minimal because of the research and development costs it would entail.

Other food-borne viruses causing gastroenteritis are Norwalk agent (Kapikan *et al.*, 1972), the cause of winter vomiting disease, now classified with similar viruses as a small round structured virus (SRSV), caliciviruses, astroviruses, and small round viruses (SRV). In the absence of bacterial pathogens the cause of food-related gastroenteritis may be assumed to be infection by SRSV if the clinical picture is similar to the pattern described by Kaplan and colleagues (1982). Because the diagnosis of infection by these viruses depends on electron microscopy or the amplification of their nucleic acid by the polymerase chain reaction (PCR), they are certainly underdiagnosed. Nevertheless, strict application of hygienic food handling methods, including close control of the health of food handlers, would reduce the incidence of viral and other forms of infective gastroenteritis.

# References

Byrd, J.J., Huai-shu, X.U. and Colwell, R.R. (1991). Viable but non-culturable bacteria in drinking water. *Applied and Environmental Microbiology* **57**, 875–878.

Chatterjee, B.D. (1982). In *Microbiology* (A.I Braude, ed.), p. 357. W.B. Saunders, Philadelphia.

Cholera Working Group, International Centre for Diarrhoea Diseases Research (1993). Large epidemic of cholera-like disease in Bangladesh caused by *Vibrio cholera* O139 synonym Bengal. *Lancet* **342**, 387–390.

Communicable Disease Report (1994). Salmonella in Humans, England and Wales: quarterly report. *Communicable Disease Report* **4**(43), 207.

Communicable Disease Report (1996). Other gastrointestinal tract infections in England and Wales: laboratory reports weeks 49–52/96. *Communicable Disease Report* **6**(2), 11.

Department of Health (1988). *Salmonella and Raw Eggs*. Department of Health, London (PL/CO(88)9).

Epstein, P.R. (1992). Cholera and the environment. *Lancet* **342**, 1167–1168.

Epstein, P.R., Ford, R.E. and Colwell, R.R. (1993). Marine ecosystems. *Lancet* **342**, 1216–1219

Gilbert, R.J., Stringer, M.F. and Peace, T.C. (1974). The survival and growth of *Bacillus cereus* in boiled and fried rice in relation to outbreaks of food poisoning. *Journal of Hygiene*, Cambridge **73**, 433–444.

Hudson, S.J., Lightfoot, N.F., Coulson, J.C. *et al.* (1991). Jackdaws and magpies as vectors of milkborne human campylobacter infection. *Epidemiology and Infection* **107**, 363–372.

Kapikian, A.Z., Wyatt, R.G., Dolin, R. *et al.* (1972). Visualization by immune electron microscopy of a 27-nm particle associated with acute infectious nonbacterial gastroenteritis. *Journal of Virology* **10**, 1075–1081.

Kaplan, J.E., Feldman, R., Campbell, D.S. *et al.* (1982). The frequency of a Norwalk-like pattern of illness in outbreaks of acute gastro-enteritis. *American Journal of Public Health* **76**, 1329–1332.

Levine,. M.M. and Kaper, J.B. (1993). Live oral vaccines against cholera: an update. *Vaccine* **11**, 207–212.

Nalin, D.R. and McLaughlin, J. (1977). Colonization of *Ascaris lumbricoides* by *V. cholerae*. *Journal of Parasitology* **62**, 839–841.

Pearson, A.D. and Healing, T.D. (1992). The surveillance and control of campylobacter infection. *Communicable Disease Report Review* **2**, R133–R139.

Philander, S.G. (1990). *El Niño, La Niña, and the Southern Oscillation*. Academic Press, London.

Rollins, D.M. and Colwell, R.R. (1986). Viable but non-culturable stage of *C. jejuni* and its role in survival in the natural aquatic environment. *Applied and Environmental Microbiology* **52**, 531–538.

Sebald, M. and Véron, M. (1963). Teneur en bases de l'ADN et classification des vibrions. *Annales de l'Institut Pasteur* **105**, 897–910.

Suharyono, Simanjuntak, C., Wetham, N. *et al.* (1992). Immunogenicity of single-dose live oral cholera vaccine CVD103-HgR in 5–9-year-old Indonesian children. *Lancet* **340**, 689–694

Swerdlow, D.L. and Ries, A.A. (1993). *Vibrio cholera* non-O1 – the eighth pandemic? *Lancet* **342**, 382–383.

# Chapter 8

# Infections caused by herpesviruses

The herpesviruses are members of a sizeable group of large viruses with diameters ranging from 85 to 110 nm. Their genomes, of linear double-stranded DNA, specify many proteins, including some with enzymic activity necessary for the replication of the virus. The specific inhibition of such virus-coded products offers a rational path to chemotherapy of infection by herpesviruses; this, indeed, is what the drug acyclovir is able to do in certain infections by herpesviruses. After entry into infected cells it is phosphorylated and the resulting acyclovir triphosphate inhibits the herpes-specific DNA polymerase, thus preventing continued synthesis of viral DNA. Acyclovir is effective against herpes simplex and varicella-zoster viruses, but has no activity against normal cellular processes.

Herpesviruses cause a variety of diseases in many vertebrate species. Many of them, for example the cytomegaloviruses, are highly species specific. During the primary infection, herpesviruses have a strong tendency to become latent, with subsequent reactivation and recurrent disease. Herpesviruses, both of animals and humans, have predilections for certain types of cell, and this has been used as a convenient, but not necessarily precise, method of classifying them. The $\alpha$ herpesviruses (e.g. herpes simplex virus) have a short reproductive cycle, and spread rapidly within infected cell cultures. Human viruses of this group are infectious, experimentally, in other species such as rabbits and mice. *In vivo* they enter latency mainly, but not exclusively, in sensory ganglion cells. The $\beta$ herpesviruses (e.g. cytomegaloviruses) have a restricted host range and replicate slowly in cell cultures, but only in cells of the species which they infect naturally. The $\gamma$ herpesviruses (e.g. EB virus) replicate in lymphoblastoid cells, being specific for either T or B cells. Under appropriate circumstances they may cause lytic infections also, in epithelioid and fibroblastic cells.

There is generally little, if any, serological relationship between different members of the groups. Eight herpesviruses have been described which infect humans. They are distinguished in the literature by numbers, for example human herpesvirus (HHV) 1, etc.; although some have names which predate the numbers. However, HHV1 and HHV2 (types 1 and 2 herpes simplex virus), which cause among the most obvious, but not necessarily the most frequent, herpesvirus infection of humans, share enough antigens to cross react in serological tests.

## HHV1

Probably most type 1 infections are acquired in infancy from a relative or carer with cold sores who is either ignorant or careless of the infectious nature of the lesions. Some primary infections are symptomless, but many present, typically, as acute stomatitis. Latency is a very probable sequel of the primary infection. The latent virus is resident – integrated in the genome of the host cells – in anatomically appropriate neural ganglion cells. Primary infection of the area innervated by the facial nerve (i.e. the great majority of type 1 infections) leads to latent infection of cells in the Gasserian ganglion, whereas type 2 infections – mainly genital – become latent in the presacral ganglion. The factors controlling recurrent attacks are ill-understood. Virus, possibly continually released from infected ganglion cells, is carried to the skin by axonal flow in the nerve fibres. Because cold sores tend to occur when the skin and mucous membranes innervated by branches of the facial nerve are damaged locally by a variety of mechanisms – shaving, repeated irritation of wet skin produced by a common cold, or by fever, or physiological changes such as those associated with menstruation, or by exposure to ultraviolet irradiation – local protective mechanisms in the skin are possibly so deranged that the virus, instead of being neutralized, is allowed to multiply, with the production of the typical lesions of herpes simplex. The presence of even substantial amounts of neutralizing antibody in the infected person's circulation is unable to prevent recurrent attacks of herpes, which suggests strongly that the intracellular situation of the virus protects it. Both HHV1 and HHV2 may be secreted in appropriate body fluids by symptom-free, latently infected subjects. Genital infections with type 1 herpes simplex virus (a minority of such infections) are said to be generally less severe clinically, and less likely to recur than type 2 infections.

## HHV2

The very wide currency of type 2 infections follows from the increased circulation of the virus in the 1960s (and subsequently) when the introduction of 'the pill' ushered in the so-called sexual revolution. Before the pill, sexual activity outside marriage was no doubt frequent even in developed industrial societies, but tended to be covert. The availability of oral contraception allowed women to control their own fertility, and sexual activity became freer and more open. With the onus of preventing pregnancy in pre- and extramarital sexual encounters transferred to women, men increasingly stopped using condoms, exposing their partners and themselves to the risk of sexually transmitted infections. This, combined with enthusiastic promiscuity, common among both sexes and all sexual orientations, established a social environment in which sexually transmitted diseases could flourish. And they did, with genital herpes among the leaders. In 1973 it was estimated, because herpes infections were (and are) not notifiable, that in the UK, Europe and the USA there were about half a million new cases of genital herpes annually (Nahmias *et al.*, 1973).

## HHV3

HHV3 (varicella-zoster virus) which causes chickenpox and zoster (shingles) is also neurotropic and an $\alpha$ herpesvirus. Primary infections cause chickenpox, a disease almost entirely of childhood. The latent virus is integrated in cells of both motor and sensory nerves. Zoster presents as a vesicular rash involving part or the whole of one or more dermatomes and is usually preceded by paraesthesiae in the affected dermatome(s). Why particular dermatomes should be implicated in the emergence of the virus from latency is unknown. Full-blown zoster is, with very few exceptions, extremely painful. Since most children have chickenpox, most of the adult population is at risk of developing zoster. Immunity to the virus is primarily cell mediated. Most cases of zoster occur later in life when the the the efficiency of the immune system is often diminished. Although zoster is generally a disease of advancing age, children with impaired cell-mediated immunity are liable to be affected by it. When a pregnant woman develops zoster close to term, the fetus is likely to be infected and to develop clinically severe chickenpox in the neonatal period. Intrauterine infection in the earlier stages of pregnancy is more likely to lead to the death of the fetus.

## HHV4

The influence of environment on epidemiology is shown particularly well by the different behaviour of Epstein–Barr (EB) virus – HHV4 – in economically developed communities and populations in developing countries. These differences are especially notable in certain tropical environments. EB virus, the causative agent of infectious mononucleosis, was originally demonstrated in lymphoblasts of Burkitt's lymphoma (Epstein et al., 1964). The aetiological relationship between the virus and infectious mononucleosis was established serendipitously when the serum of a laboratory worker, which was used as a negative control in experiments with Burkitt's lymphoma, was found to be positive when she returned to work after recovering from infectious mononucleosis (Henle et al., 1968).

In western, temperate-climate societies, infectious mononucleosis in economically better-off groups is predominantly a disease of adolescents and young adults. The transmission of infection is thought to depend on close contact, especially of mucous membranes, naming it a so-called 'kissing disease' (Hoagland, 1967). In developing countries, however, where there is often much poverty and deprivation – malnutrition, overcrowding, and generally unhygienic conditions (Evans, 1974) – infection occurs at a much younger age, often with little immediately obvious clinical consequence. This pattern of infection can be seen in Britain in nurseries (Pereira et al., 1969), and among other aggregations of very young children, where subclinical infection is common, as shown by antibody surveys. EB virus is excreted by the pharyngeal mucosa, and the high incidence of infection in nurseries and similar situations suggests that dissemination of virus from patients' mouths by aerosol may be a factor in its spread, although in children of this age group more direct transfer of saliva from one to another is common.

An important diagnostic feature of infectious mononucleosis is the appearance in the blood stream, often transiently, of morphologically altered mononuclear cells resembling lymphoblasts; and EB virus can be recovered from B lymphocytes of patients in the acute stage of the disease (Rocchi et al., 1977). It is therefore classified as a $\gamma$ herpesvirus. It is in this type of cell that latent infection with EB virus occurs. This is significant, because Burkitt's lymphomas are monoclonal, of B lymphocyte lineage.

Although infectious mononucleosis and serum antibody to EB virus are ubiquitous, and patients with Burkitt's lymphoma have high concentrations of antibody, the neoplasm in endemic form is confined to regions of very warm, humid climate which are holoendemic for malaria, such as may be found in tropical Africa and Papua New Guinea. Scattered cases of Burkitt's lymphoma occur in many other, non-malarious, parts of the world. In about half the cases of each sort there is a similar genomic abnormality – a translocation between chromosomes 8 and 14. The mechanism by which a cell latently infected by EB virus, i.e. carrying the virus genome integrated in its own genome, is transformed into a neoplastic cell is not known. However, a reasonable supposition is that some infected children (perhaps with another genomic abnormality which would otherwise be of no great significance) are so immunocompromised by their heavy load of malarial parasites that the signs of virus activity are no longer confined to the expression of certain virus antigens at the cell surface, but the integrated virus is now able to replicate to a morphologically recognizable form, and at the same time makes, or initiates, a signal, or a series of signals, to set the neoplastic process going. This does not, however, offer much, if any, insight into the pathogenesis of Burkitt's lymphoma in subjects lacking the chromosomal transloca-tion mentioned above. Nevertheless, a possible result of global warming could be the return to Britain of endemic malaria, the last indigenous case of which was reported in 1957. The vectors of malaria parasites are anopheline mosquitoes. Five species of *Anopheles* are present in the country, and a sustained, unspectacular rise in mean temperature of a mere degree Celsius would facilitate a rapid increase in mosquito populations. The importance of concomitant malaria in the pathogenesis of Burkitt's lymphoma is shown by the virtual disappearance of the condition from such subtropical areas as the northern part of KwaZulu-Natal where malaria has been controlled. Holoendemic malaria would be an unlikely development in Britain and the rest of Europe, but a warmer climate might well alter social interactions – especially of families with very young children – thus leading to infection with EB virus at a much younger age than is common at present.

High concentrations of antibody against EB virus are also present in the serum of patients in East Africa (Kenya) and south China suffering from nasopharyngeal carcinoma. The carcinoma generally occurs in African adults between the ages of 20 and 50 with a ratio of males to females of 2:1 and an incidence rate of about 1 per 100 000. In parts of Africa children and adolescents may also develop the condition. In south China, however, the rate is about 10 per 100 000 (and in boat dwellers 16 per 100 000). In ethnic Chinese with roots in south China the rate is high wherever they live: in Singapore it is about 29 per 100 000.

Since infection with EB virus is virtually universal, it would be injudicious to suggest an aetiological relationship between virus and neoplasm were it not for two factors:

1. The concentrations of antiviral antibody in persons with the carcinoma are much greater than those found in non-

carcinomatous subjects at a similar period after infection with the virus.
2. The presence of EB virus DNA in the nuclei of nasopharyngeal cancer cells.

Several environmental risk factors – seemingly not active in the absence of infection with EB virus – have been implicated: exposure to fumes, chemicals and smoke, and the consumption of salt-cured fish. For ethnic Chinese there appears also to be a genetic factor which acts as a multiplier of risk. One must assume that, if two such different neoplasms as Burkitt's lymphoma and nasopharyngeal carcinoma depend in some way on the presence in their cells of the genome of EB virus, either the oncogenic triggers are sufficiently disparate to account for the different types of malignancy which result, or EB virus is able to become latent in epithelial as well as lymphoid cells.

The oncogenic potential of EB virus has apparently not yet been fully disclosed. For some time a relationship between Hodgkin's disease and previous infection with EB virus has been suspected. EB virus has been associated with malignancy – but not necessarily causally – for many years (Johanssen et al., 1970). More recently, ample evidence has been offered of EB-virus DNA in the nuclei, and EB-virus antigens at the surface of Hodgkin and Reed-Sternberg cells – the pathognomonic cells of Hodgkin's lymphoma. Some workers doubt whether the virus is actually oncogenic and not simply present in the cells as a passenger (Pallesen et al., 1991; O'Grady et al., 1994). The doubt arises because the antigen in question – latent membrane protein (LMP-1) – is not expressed in all Hodgkin's tumours.

Given the propensity of herpesviruses to be integrated in infected host cells, it is not surprising that a few of them may, in ways at present unknown, promote malignancy in some infected cells. That the malignancies recognized to date are as different as Burkitt's lymphoma, nasopharyngeal carcinoma, Hodgkin's disease and Kaposi's sarcoma (see below), suggests either that more than one pathway may exist to immortalization of cells, or that there is, for each malignancy, an external environmental factor, or a factor resident in the cells, which differs from that in the others, and leads to a different type of cancer.

## HHV5

Human cytomegalovirus, a $\beta$ herpesvirus, is similar to viruses which have been identified in many vertebrate species. The viruses are highly species specific, and can be isolated and cultivated only in cells of the appropriate host species. Intrauterine infection of the fetus may occur, most commonly during the second and third trimesters of pregnancy (Alford *et al.*, 1980). If the infection occurs early in the pregnancy the infant is likely to show a very severe form of cytomegalic disease. Horizontal infection may occur at any age after birth, and may be followed by prolonged periods of excretion of the virus. This is especially so when very young children are infected – they may continue to excrete virus for several years. In much of the world, although only about 1% of fetuses are infected, about 10% of such infants show signs of cytomegalic inclusion disease. Largely because of the very large number of births cytomegalovirus infection is a, if not the, major cause of congenital infection. It is likely to cause serious defects in the baby, but there is some doubt as to whether congenital infection is more likely to occur when the mother suffers a primary infection during her pregnancy, or when she experiences a reactivation infection. Typical cellular lesions of cytomegalic inclusion disease – swollen cells with enlarged nuclei containing inclusions – can be found in many organs. Antibody surveys in various parts of the world have shown an increasing prevalence of infection with increasing age.

The virus can be isolated from leucocytes during the lifetime of the infected person. It can thus be transmitted by blood transfusion; but infection usually depends on the patient receiving many transfusions from many different donors. Infection is frequent after kidney transplantation from antibody-positive donors to antibody-negative recipients. The fact that such a recipient undergoes seroconversion does not necessarily mean that symptomatic disease will occur, or that – if it does – it will be severe. Heart transplantation is commonly followed by seroconversion, but it is often unclear whether this is directly referable to the transplanted organ or to the large volumes of donor blood to which the recipient is exposed during the course of surgery. When the infection is acquired at any period after birth, symptoms occur more commonly in adults than in children. It has been suggested that seronegative subjects should be transfused only with seronegative blood; but because of the increased likelihood of infection in organ donors, and the shortage of organ donations, ensuring that transplants to susceptible patients are made only from seronegative donors would be well-nigh impossible.

Asymptomatic infants and children may excrete large amounts of virus in urine and saliva. Since naturally occurring, extrauterine infection appears to depend on close individual contact, for example between children, or between children and adults caring for them, or even between susceptible (seronegative) subjects and toys or other objects contaminated with the saliva of a virus-excreting baby, nurseries and day-care facilities may provide suitable environments for the transmission of infection. Although much earlier work indicated that congenital and perinatal infections were more common among the financially less well off in industrialized societies (Epstein *et al.*, 1964), later investigations have suggested that, with an increase in breast feeding among women of social groups A, B, and possibly C1, there may be a greater chance of perinatal infection of their infants. Also because an increased proportion of such women go out to work, day-care arrangements will also influence the epidemiology of cytomegalovirus infection in this segment of society (Stagno and Cloud, 1994).

Primary infection with cytomegalovirus may cause a glandular fever syndrome clinically very similar to infectious mononucleosis. The diagnosis is suggested by a persistently negative Paul-Bunnell test or by the absence of IgM specific for EB virus.

Reactivated cytomegalovirus frequently appears in the uterine cervix, and can be isolated from the semen of infected men. Sexual transmission of the virus is thus possible, as is infection of the infant during parturition.

The distribution of cytomegalovirus is worldwide but, as with measles, the epidemiology of infection differs under different environmental conditions. In industrially developed countries of the western world more than half the adults are infected by age 50. According to Tobin (1983), in women of child-bearing age, the incidence of antibody varies from 40 to about 60% in most temperate climates. Many babies are thus born with ample passive immunity which diminishes significantly in the first 6 months of life. In southern India, however, antibody to cytomegalovirus – measured by complement fixation tests – was present in 80% of children by age 4; there was a very high prevalence in several Melanesian populations; while in Nova Scotia only three out of 548 children excreted the virus in their urine (Christie, 1987). Unlike the situation in Europe and the USA where, in general, the incidence of antibody to cytomegalovirus increases with increasing age in a population (Stern, 1968), in those parts of the world, especially Africa, South America and much of Asia, which are economically under-developed, deficient in hygiene, and where there is a tendency to live communally, infection, as shown by the age of acquisition of antibody, occurs early in life. In Papua New Guinea, the Solomon Islands and Vanuatu, for example, a high proportion of small samples of sera contained antibody by age 4 years, and by the age of about 15 years, there was a high incidence in large samples (Long *et al.*, 1997).

## HHV6

HHV6 was discovered in 1986 (Salahuddin *et al.*, 1986), and thought to be associated with B-cell tumours. Its subsequent isolation from normal tissues (Lusso *et al.*, 1987) pointed to its being a passenger in lymphoid tumours. It infects young children, causing exanthem subitum (Yamanishi *et al.*, 1988), a normally self-limiting condition in which the infected infant develops a high fever for a few days, which is followed by a rash as the fever abates. Liver function tests are often abnormal, and there may be lymphadeno-pathy, and perhaps encephalitis. Antibody to the virus is widely prevalent in the population (Knowles and Gardner, 1988). After the waning of passively conferred maternal immunity, most children are infected by the age of 2 years. The source of infection is unclear, but the virus is present in the saliva of most adults. This is a possible route of infection from mother to infant. The virus remains in the body when the clinical condition resolves, either as a persistent or a latent infection. It has been associated with hepatitis (Dubedat and Kappagoda, 1989). Although there was originally doubt about the classification of HHV6, it is now classified as a $\beta$ herpesvirus.

## HHV7

This virus, first isolated from a healthy person (Frenkel *et al.*, 1990), is a $\beta$ herpesvirus, related to, but different from, HHV5 (human cytomegalovirus) and HHV6 (Berneman *et al.*, 1992). In cultures of appropriate human cells it forms syncytia which are inhibited by specific antibody. A test based on this phenomenon (Secchiero *et al.*, 1994) found antibody in serum samples from 30 normal adults, as well as in a few persons with AIDS, chronic fatigue syndrome, and chronic lymphatic leukaemia; this suggests that it may well be a normally non-pathogenic passenger virus widely disseminated in humans.

## HHV8

Kaposi's sarcoma has for some years been thought to be related to a herpesvirus (Giraldo *et al.*, 1972). Firm evidence was lacking, but the existence of the sarcoma in about 40% of homosexual men with AIDS, and its extreme rarity in haemophiliacs with AIDS, suggested that it might be not only infectious, but sexually transmitted (Beral *et al.*, 1990). In 1994 herpes-like DNA sequences were demonstrated in Kaposi's sarcoma from patients with AIDS (Chang *et al.*, 1994). Subsequently, about three-quarters of patients infected with HIV, in whose blood the presence of a herpesvirus (dubbed HHV8) was detected, developed Kaposi's sarcoma within 5 years (Whitby *et al.*, 1995). A latently infected line of B cells from a lymphomatous ascites tumour was treated with phorbol esters, leading to active production of the latent virus, and the presence of fully formed herpes virions in the cells (Renne *et al.*, 1996). This allowed the virus to be characterized (Moore *et al.*, 1996). It resembled EB virus in its tissue tropism more closely than any of the other human herpesviruses. It is probably a γ virus. Whether Kaposi's sarcoma in patients infected with HIV results from reactivation of latent HHV8 or from infection with the virus at the same time and by the same route as their infection with HIV is open to question. This, of course, throws no light on the origin of the virus in sporadic cases of Kaposi's sarcoma in elderly Caucasians, a minority of whom are females.

# References

Alford, C.A., Stagno, S., Pass, R.F. and Huang, E-S. (1990). In *The Human Herpesviruses: An Interdisciplinary perspective* (A.J. Nahmias, W.R. Dowdle, and R.F. Schinazi (eds). Elsevier, New York.

Beral, V., Peterman, T.A., Berkelman, R.L. and Jaffe, H.C.W. (1990). Kaposi's sarcoma among persons with AIDS: a sexually transmitted infection? *Lancet* **335**, 123–128.

Berneman, Z.N., Ablashi, D.V., Li, G., *et al.* (1992). Human herpesvirus 7 is a T-lymphotropic virus and is related to, but significantly different from Human herpesvirus 6 and human cytomegalovirus. *Proceedings of the National Academy of Science of the USA* **89**, 10552–10556.

Chang, Y., Cesarman, E., Pessin, M.S. *et al.* (1994). Identification of herpes-like DNA sequences in AIDS-associated Kaposi's sarcoma. *Science* **266**, 1865–1869.

Christie, A.B. (1987). Quoting several authors. In *Infectious Diseases*, 4th ed. Churchill Livingstone, Edinburgh.

Dubedat S. & Kappagoda, N. (1989). Hepatitis due to human herpesvirus 6. *Lancet* **ii**, 1463–1464.

Epstein, M.A., Achong, B.G. and Barr, Y.M. (1964). Virus particles in cultured lymphoblasts from Burkitt's lymphoma. *Lancet* **i**, 702-703.

Evans, A.S. (1974). The history of infectious mononucleosis. *American Journal of Medical Science* **267**, 189–195.

Frenkel, N., Schirmer, E.C., Wyeth, L.S. *et al.* (1990). Isolation of a new herpesvirus from human CD4$^+$ T cells. *Proceedings of the National Academy of Science of the USA* **87**, 748–752.

Giraldo, G., Beth, E. and Hagenau, F. (1972). Herpes-type virus particles in tissue culture of Kaposi's sarcoma from different geographic regions. *Journal of the National Cancer Institute* **49**, 1509–1526.

Henle, G., Henle, W. and Diehl, V. (1968). Relation of Burkitt's tumour-associated herpes-type virus to infectious mononucleosis. *Proceedings of the National Academy of Science of the USA* **59**, 94–101.

Hoagland, R.J. (1967). *Infectious Mononucleosis*. Grune & Stratton, New York.

Johansson, B., Klein, G., Henle, W. and Henle, G. (1970). Epstein–Barr virus (EBV)-associated antibody patterns in malignant lymphoma and leukemia. *International Journal of Cancer* **6**, 450–462.

Knowles, W.A. and Gardner, S.D. (1988). High prevalence of antibody to human herpesvirus-6 and seroconversion associated with rash in two infants. *Lancet* **ii**, 912–913.

Long, D.J., Garruto, R.M. and Gajdusek, D.C. (1977). Early acquisition of cytomegalovirus and Epstein-Barr antibodies. *American Journal of Epidemiology* **105**, 480–487.

Lusso, P., Salahuddin, S.Z., Ablashi, D.V. *et al.* (1987). Diverse tropism of human B-lymphotropic virus (HHV-6). *Lancet* **ii**, 743–744.

Moore, P.S., Gao, S-H., Dumingnez, G. *et al.* (1996). Primary characterization of a herpesvirus agent associated with Kaposi's sarcoma. *Journal of Virology* **70**, 549–558.

Nahmias, A.J., von Reyn, C.F. Josey, W.E. *et al.* (1973). Genital herpes simplex infection and gonorrhoea: association and analogies. *British Journal of Venereal Disease* **49**, 306–309.

O'Grady J., Stewart, S., Elton, R.A. and Krajewski, A.S. (1994). Epstein–Barr virus in Hodgkin's disease and site of origin of tumour. *Lancet* **343**, 265–266.

Pallesen, G., Hamilton-Dutoit, S.J., Rowe, M. and Young, L.S. (1991). Expression of Epstein–Barr virus latent gene products in tumour cells of Hodgkin's disease. *Lancet* **337**, 320–322.

Pereira, M.S., Blake, J.M. and Macrae, A.D. (1969). EB antibody at different ages. *British Medical Journal* **iv**, 526–527.

Renne, R., Zhong, W., Herndier, B. *et al.* (1996). Lytic growth of Kaposi's sarcoma-associated herpesvirus (human herpesvirus 8) in culture. *Nature Medicine* **3**, 342–346.

Rocchi, G., de Felici, A., Ragona, G. and Heinz, A. (1977). Quantitative evaluation of Epstein–Barr-virus-infected peripheral blood leukocytes in infectious mononucleosis. *New England Journal of Medicine* **296**, 132–134.

Salahuddin, S.Z., Ablasbi, D.V., Markham, P.D. *et al.* (1986). Isolation of a new virus (HBLV), in patients with lymphoproliferative disorders. *Science* **234**, 596–601.

Secchiero, P., Berneman, Z.N., Gallo, R.C. and Lusso, P. (1994). Biological and molecular characteristics of HHV7: *in vitro* growth optimization and development of a syncytia inhibition test. *Virology* **202**, 506–512.

Stagno, S. and Cloud, G.A. (1994). Working parents: the impact of day care and breast-feeding on cytomegalovirus infection in offspring. *Proceedings of the National Academy of Science of the USA* **91**, 2384–2389.

Stern, H. (1968). Isolation of cytomegalovirus and clinical manifestations of infection at different ages. *British Medical Journal* **i**, 665–669.

Tobin, J.O'H. (1983). *Cytomegalovirus infection*. Oxford Textbook of Medicine (D.J.

Weatherall, J.G.G. Ledingham and D.A. Warrell, eds) p 5.65. Oxford University Press, Oxford.

Whitby, D., Howard, M.R., Tenant-Flowers, M. *et al.* (1995). Detection of Kaposi sarcoma associated herpesvirus in peripheral blood of HIV-infected individuals and progression to Kaposi's sarcoma. *Lancet* **346**, 799–802.

Yamanishi, K., Okuno, T., Shiraki, K. *et al.* (1988). Identification of human herpesvirus-6 as a causal agent for exanthem subitum. *Lancet* **i**, 1065–1067.

# Chapter 9

# Vector-borne bacterial infections

Several important infections are caused by bacteria which depend on arthropod vectors both for their transmission and their maintenance in animal reservoirs. This chapter considers diseases caused by three different genera. Infection of humans by these pathogens is clearly related to environmental factors, changes in which might well be accompanied by altered disease incidences. The most widely known of these diseases is probably bubonic plague, caused by the bacterium *Yersinia pestis* which is transmitted from infected rodents to other hosts, including man, by fleas. Rickettsioses include a range of, mostly, zoonotic diseases transmitted by the bites of a host of arthropods – lice, ticks, mites and fleas; at least one – Q fever – is spread by the aerial route. Historically, the most important has been typhus, transmitted by lice and fleas. It has, in its time, killed hundreds of thousands of people in epidemic outbreaks. Lyme disease is a bacterial infection transmitted by ticks. Although some of its signs and symptoms were first described in 1910, Lyme disease is regarded as an emerging disease, for reasons to be discussed later. It appears to be of worldwide distribution with a high but not precisely known prevalence. It has been pointed out (Morse and Schluederberg, 1990) that the majority of emerging infectious diseases, whatever their causes, are zoonoses and 'often follow ecological changes caused by human activities such as agriculture, agricultural change, migration, urbanization, deforestation or dam building'.

## Plague

Plague is primarily an enzootic infection of burrowing colonial rodents such as the susliks and tarbagans of Far East Russia, gerbils which are endemic in parts of the Kalahari desert and the semi-arid Karroo of South Africa, and ground squirrels in the western USA. This is sylvatic plague, in which the infection is spread within burrows by the bites of fleas which have become infected by taking a blood meal from an infected inhabitant. The bacteria multiply in the proventriculus and stomach of the infected flea; its host either recovers from the infection or dies. If it dies, the flea transfers itself to a living host. When it next attempts to take a meal the blood it ingests is confined to the oesophagus because the proventriculus is now blocked by the growth of *Y. pestis* acquired from its previous host. The flea continues sucking blood until its grossly stretched oesophagus contracts, forcing blood and bacteria back into the host animal, thus transmitting the infection.

Even a 'new' infectious agent seldom kills 100% of the animals (or people) it infects. Myxomatosis virus, for example, entirely unknown to Australian rabbits before 1950, although very lethal, had an overall kill rate of less than 100% in the first year or so of the epizooty. It was not much less than 100%, but enough individuals survived, to breed and, in the course of several years, to re-establish the population.

When epizootic plague strikes a rodent colony some burrows may be wiped out, but not every rodent in every burrow dies. Fleas, and the bacteria they carry, have been shown to survive in burrows for several months in the absence of suitable blood meals. As the rodent colony reconstitutes itself, it contains enough susceptible animals to support the enzootic presence of *Y. pestis*. In semi-arid regions rains occur infrequently, but when they do, they greatly increase food supplies, and are commonly followed by a large expansion of the rodent population, virtually the whole of which, lacking immunity, is susceptible to infection with *Y. pestis*. Under these conditions enzootic infection rapidly becomes epizootic. This greatly increases the chance of spread beyond the colony in the period before the epizooty markedly reduces the size of the population once again. Experience has shown that human outbreaks of plague are preceded by the die-off of wild-rodent colonies 6–12 months earlier and accompanied by a reduction in numbers of domestic rodents (Davis, 1948).

Despite their normal predilection for a particular host species, so-called blocked fleas become very hungry and will take blood meals from any available warm-blooded host, including man. Human populations are involved in epidemic outbreaks either, rarely, by direct contact with infected colonial rodents or, more usually, when the infection has been transferred from a sylvatic focus to a rodent species which is at home with humans. In South Africa, for example, where the ecology of plague has been extensively studied (Davis, 1948), the main sylvatic hosts are gerbils, especially *Tatera brantsi* in the Kalahari Desert and the drier parts of the north-west Cape Province and the Orange Free State, and *Desmodillus auricularis* in the southerly Little Karroo; although other colonial rodents may also be implicated. Migrant blocked fleas tend to transfer to the multimammate mouse (*Mastomys natalensis*) which, in rural areas, forages abroad where it may meet infected fleas, and also inhabits huts and other dwellings where fleas may have the opportunity to attempt to feed on humans. In urban areas adjacent to sylvatic foci (e.g. in the Port Elizabeth outbreak of 1938), the house rat, *Rattus rattus*, carries the infection into close proximity to human beings. Where *R. rattus* populations declined, as in parts of India, human cases of plague became fewer and fewer, but other rodents became involved, such as *Bandicota bengalensis* in Bombay and Calcutta. Increased numbers of *R. rattus*, however, may well be followed by epidemic plague in human populations (see below).

Sylvatic plague exists, and indeed prospers, among burrowing rodents in semi-arid parts of the world in addition to South Africa: the prairies of the American West, the pampas of South America, the steppes of Far Eastern Russia and Manchuria. Any extension of such areas which results from major climatic changes may be expected to be followed by the extension of the endemicity of their burrowing rodents, and with it, of foci of sylvatic plague. Ecological studies have suggested that short of wholesale slaughter of all the rodent colonies in a plague focus, the risk of infection could not readily be eradicated. However, the distribution of insecticides within burrows may reduce the incidence of epizootic sylvatic plague by reducing flea populations, thus diminishing the likelihood of overspill to intermediary populations of rodents and hence the risk of both sporadic and epidemic plague in humans.

The pneumonic form is an important but epidemiologically less frequent clinical type of plague. The case fatality rate of untreated bubonic plague varies from 30–70%. Pneumonic plague is considerably more lethal. Before effective treatment by broad-spectrum antibiotics was introduced in the 1950s, very few patients survived. The index case or cases of pneumonic plague can acquire the infection by direct contact with a sylvatic focus of infection, as appears to have happened in Manchuria in 1910 during an unskilled free-for-all hunting of marmots for their fur-bearing skins; but most pneumonic plague occurs as secondary pneumonia in patients with bubonic plague. The epidemic spread of the pneumonic form requires extremely cold weather and severe overcrowding of dwellings. In an established outbreak, mortality may be great. In the Manchurian epidemic of 1910–11 the overall case fatality rate was very high – in some centres actually reaching 100%. Almost 60 000 died between September 1910 and April 1911, a total helped on not only by the weather and large collections of overcrowded people, but also by the fact that the infection was spread for long distances by the railways (Twigg, 1984a). A rather similar epidemic picture – aided by the upheaval of war – emerged during the second Manchurian epidemic 10 years later. Both episodes clearly indicate the potential importance of human incursions into, and alteration of, the environment. Shrewsbury's opinion, as a historian of plague in Britain, that pneumonic plague never occurs in the absence of bubonic plague (Shrewsbury, 1971) is clearly untenable as a generalization, but may well be correct in the context of Great Britain. Should the global alteration of climate cause Britain to become warmer and drier, changes in rodent populations could be expected. Nevertheless even if *Y. pestis* was introduced, the behaviour of the Suffolk epizooty in the years before the First World War (Twigg, 1984b) suggests that enzootic plague, at least, would be an unlikely problem; however, there could be no certainty about other infections dependent on rodent reservoirs.

Clearly, while foci of sylvatic plague remain in existence, nearby domestic and peridomestic environments which attract rats and other potential intermediary species of rodents will continue to keep human populations at risk of epidemic outbreaks of plague. Environments of this sort, in which people live crowded together in makeshift hovels with, at best, rudimentary sanitary arrangements, exist in Africa and the Indian subcontinent close to old-established plague foci. After two recent outbreaks of plague in India, the government appointed a Technical Advisory Committee to report on them. The Committee's Report, briefly summarized (Technical Advisory Committee, 1995), clearly shows that the outbreaks were investigated thoroughly, and that, despite the rapidity with which they were controlled, there were serious gaps in India's defences against epidemic infectious diseases. Similar gaps probably exist elsewhere.

In August 1994 an outbreak of bubonic plague in the district of Beed in Maharashtra State followed a severe flea nuisance and the deaths of numbers of rats. Although no isolations of *Y. pestis* were made at the time, unmistakable antigens of the organism were identified in several pools of fleas collected in the area of the most heavily infected village in October. In September 1994 in Surat, a city in the neighbouring State of Gujarat, an acute pneumonic disease occurred in increasing numbers, and an outbreak of pneumonic plague was diagnosed. Both outbreaks were contained rapidly, but in neither was the aetiological agent identified at the time, although laboratory confirmations were made later. There was a 'cascade of eco-epidemiological evidence' about the origins of the outbreaks. In September 1993 there was an earthquake which disturbed 'the pre-existing equilibrium between wild and domestic rodents and fleas'. This was followed by a notable increase in populations of *Rattus rattus* (the house rat), the flea nuisance of August, and ratfalls which preceded the appearance of buboes in the human population. The origins of the pneumonic plague in Surat were less clear. There is no certainty of antecedent bubonic plague, but there were environmental disturbances – flooding of a local river and crowds of people at a religious festival – which may have contributed. However, the evidence, though weak because of the paucity of microbiological investigation, is enough to highlight the importance of altered environment in the causal chain leading to these outbreaks.

Plague, like cholera, cannot be eradicated, but can be readily controlled if infected rodents and human cases are detected early enough by epidemiological surveillance. There is, of course, a cost: effective surveillance does not come cheap. Also like cholera, the permanent control of plague depends on economic development to make hygienic housing and efficient public utilities possible; in the last analysis, the solution is not medical, but financial and engineering.

## Rickettsioses

The *Rickettsiae* are small bacteria which have lost the ability to generate their own energy requirements, and because of this they are intracellular parasites. Rickettsial infections are found worldwide. They fall into three groups. The tick-borne infections are characterized by Rocky Mountain spotted fever (most cases of which occur in the Mid-atlantic and south-east states of the USA), *fièvre boutonneuse*, and several febrile conditions known locally as tick typhuses. Various rodents and other mammals are the reservoirs of infection, but the ticks which act as vectors may also be part of the reservoir because not only do they survive the infection, but also transovarial infection of progeny is common. While feeding, the tick excretes faeces loaded with rickettsias which enter the body of the host through skin abraded by scratching provoked by the irritation caused by the tick. Because they are zoonoses, these infections are acquired through contact with the vectors, and are thus more frequent in those exposed to the appropriate environments, especially those engaged in rural work or leisure pursuits; however, it must be remembered that because dogs are commonly the source of blood meals, infected ticks may be brought into homes. Under these circumstances infection may occur when a dog's owner removes a tick from the animal without taking adequate precautions against crushing the acarid and contaminating a possibly minute blemish on a finger with the creature's juices. The period of greatest risk of infection, either in the field or elsewhere, is during late spring (when the tick feeds for a long period, and may transmit the infecting dose) and summer (when the period of feeding, and hence of transmission, is shorter).

The trend in industrially developed countries such as the USA for farmlands to be converted into suburban housing developments, and woodlands and other country areas to be used increasingly for recreation, means that more people will be at risk of infestation by ticks. Human infections can be avoided by chemical control of the vectors, but this is not a method of choice because of the ecological disturbance which would be caused by the extensive use of insecticides in woodlands and other habitats suitable for ticks. Individuals can deny access to ticks by dressing in suitably designed clothing which, because of discomfort, is not always acceptable. Because the rickettsias of this group are so deeply ensconced in their (non-human) mammalian and acarid hosts, the diseases they cause are – unlike smallpox – not susceptible to eradication.

Although its incidence today is a mere shadow of what it was a century ago, typhus is inherently the most important rickettsial disease because of its historically attested epidemic potential and high case fatality rate. For centuries it participated in the human condition. Indeed, so great was its dependence on overcrowding, filth, hunger and general deprivation, that it may truly be said to have helped shape it, especially – but by no means entirely – during times of war. It regularly accompanied armies, certainly killing more people than did the dogs of war. But even in peacetime it was active in slum quarters and as jail fever, to prevent which, British judges carried to the Bench a posy of flowers to purify the air they breathed – a custom which is now traditional.

Two types of typhus are distinguished, epidemic, which is louse borne, and endemic (or murine) which is transmitted by fleas. Human body and head lice (*Pediculus humanus*), which are infected when they feed on subjects with rickettsaemia, die within 7–10 days, but not before they have excreted faeces loaded with rickettsias. When the host scratches, the abrasion of the skin allows entry of the microbes and initiation of a new cycle of infection. Although the infective agent, *R. prowazekii*, has been isolated from ticks, it was accepted until relatively recently that epidemic typhus depended on a human–louse–human cycle of the causative agent. This suggested that it might be eradicated by eliminating the vector, because the transmitting lice do not survive the infection. After recovery from epidemic typhus, individuals may continue to be infected, asymptomatically, for many years. Perhaps because intercurrent disease or increasing age reduces their resistance, some of them develop a clinically mild condition which is, nevertheless, a form of typhus known as Brill–Zinsser disease. Lice feeding on such patients are infected and able to pass the infection on via their faeces. Sporadic cases of what was described as 'nonepidemic "epidemic" typhus' in Virginia, West Virginia, and North Carolina, were shown to be caused by *R. prowazekii*. There was strong circumstantial evidence that seven of these cases could have acquired their infections from the southern flying squirrel, *Glaucomys volans* (Duma *et al.*, 1981), a rather high proportion of which have antibody to the rickettsia, and from which *R. prowazekii* has been isolated. There may, therefore, be other non-human reservoirs of the rickettsia of epidemic typhus in other parts of the world; though such a phenomenon is not necessary to explain the survival of epidemic typhus, which surfaces from time to time in the cooler, mountainous areas of Africa – Lesuto, Rwanda, the highlands of Ethiopia – and in northern India and Afghanistan, and parts of Central and South America.

The wider importance of this is that several of these places are likely sources of migration (whether legal or illegal) to Europe or North America. The probability is that many such immigrants would be living in straitened circumstances in substandard accommodation – conditions conducive to intercurrent infection with possible activation of Brill–Zinsser disease and the consequent infection of human body lice. An increase in the incidence of lousiness in some population groups in Britain, as has occurred in the latter part of the twentieth century, combined with a significant degree of illegal immigration, could well be the basis for epidemic outbreaks of typhus. Once detected, such outbreaks could be brought under control speedily by mass treatment of affected and threatened groups with pyrethroid insecticides to rid them rapidly of lice. Several outbreaks and incipient outbreaks of epidemic typhus were controlled immediately after the Second World War by the energetic use of DDT powder, but this particular agent would be regarded as environmentally unfriendly today. Despite the relative ease with which typhus could be controlled in industrially developed countries, generalized panic promoted by scare stories in the less responsible newspapers would be very disruptive.

The endemic, and clinically milder, form of typhus is caused by infection with *R. mooseri* which has a reservoir in rats and and mice and is transmitted within the reservoir by both their lice and their fleas. Since the rat flea *Xenopsylla cheopis* will also feed on humans, transmission of murine typhus is via these fleas which, like lice, excrete the rickettsias in their faeces. Consequently, murine typhus is also a disease of poverty, crowding and dirt, likely to be prevalent in situations of continuing social deprivation.

Many years ago Zinsser (1935) wrote of the immense influence typhus has had on civilizations and human history. Despite the absence of recent large epidemic outbreaks of the disease, his book is still apposite, and should be read and digested by all – including administrators – who have an interest in public health.

## Lyme disease

In 1910 Dr Afzelius, a Swedish dermatologist, reported a condition in which a circular erythematous skin rash expanded from the site of a tick bite. He called it *erythema migrans*, and suggested that it was caused by an infection transmitted from the biting tick. Almost 40 years later another Swede reported the presence of images, which could have been those of spirochaetes, in electron micrographs of biopsies from erythema migrans. No organisms were isolated from biopsy material, but treatment of patients with penicillin was effective. Subsequently, meningitis was reported in a few patients with erythema migrans, but there was little further investigation until 1975, when there was an outbreak of a condition diagnosed as 'juvenile rheumatoid arthritis' in and around the town of Lyme in Connecticut (Steere *et al.*, 1977). This was characterized by arthritis affecting at most a few joints, and frequently only one. The condition appeared to have a predilection for the knee and in some patients was preceded by a generalized erythematous rash.

Because the outbreak occurred as a cluster of cases, mainly among children, and in summer, the investigators, suspecting that the condition was acquired during outdoor pursuits, were able to relate it to the most commonly occurring tick in the area, *Ixodes dammini* (Steere *et al.*, 1978). The spirochaete, *Borrelia burgdorferi*, was subsequently isolated from ticks (Burgdorfer *et al.*, 1982) and from patients with Lyme disease in the USA (Benach *et al.*, 1983), and erythema migrans in Europe (including Britain), where *Ixodes ricinus* is the most frequently occurring tick. Infection with *B. burgdorferi* has been reported from many countries and most continents. In the UK infected ticks have been found in the New Forest and other parts of southern England (O'Connel, 1993), and in the Scottish Highlands. Cases of erythema migrans and Lyme disease have been reported from Cambridge (Goldin *et al.*, 1978), and other parts of Britain; but the number does not seem to be great. Investigation in other parts of the country will doubtless show the infection to be widely distributed. The risk of infection is directly related to the degree of exposure to ticks, but this is modified by the incidence of infection in ticks.

To reduce the amount of farm produce, especially cereals, subject to intervention buying in terms of the European Union's Common Agricultural Policy, the British government introduced a system by which farmers 'set aside' for 1–4 years up to 10% of otherwise productive land for restoration to a state of nature – or at least a state of managed nature. For this the farmers receive a payment from the public purse and are supposed to allow public access to the 'set aside'. Most farmers in the scheme apparently opt for periods of 1 year, and use the 'set aside' as a rotational fallow. The occasional setting aside of larger areas for longer periods could lead to the formation of miniature nature reserves scattered about the country, with wildlife encouraged in a controlled sort of way, and, in terms of the 'set aside', the public being permitted access. In some of these reserves the populations of rodents will, and larger animals such as deer may, increase. In areas where *B. burgdorferi* is already present the risk of contact between humans and ticks may be expected to increase, and with it, the incidence of Lyme disease, especially if many of the visitors are town folk not previously exposed to country hazards. However, since most farmers are happy to accept the payments, but are not eager to admit the public, any increased transmission of Lyme disease or other zoonoses is likely to be more theoretical than real.

The incidence of infection in ticks in various parts of the world is far from uniform. On Shelter Island, New York, where the first isolation of the spirochaete from ticks was made, up to 100% of ticks sampled were infected. In California, where *I. pacificus* is the endemic ixodid tick, only 2% were infected. In Switzerland, up to 36% of *I. ricinus* were infected. In 17 sites in the New Forest the incidence in ticks varied from 0 to 70%; should a considerable increase in the rodent population coincide with a flush of ticks, the risks to the human population using any affected area would be increased.

Some patients investigated in Britain have been infected locally, and others abroad, including Austria and France. More than 30 000 new cases are reported annually in Germany, which may be an indication of overdiagnosis (Steere *et al.*, 1993); and 1 000 in Sweden. The disease has also been reported from Russia, China, Japan, Australia and South Africa. It is the most common bacterial infection transmitted by an arthropod in the USA; 11 000 cases were reported in 1994 – an increase of 40% over 1993 (Relman, 1995). This is probably more an indicator of increased awareness of the disease than a real increase in its incidence. In its varied manifestations, Lyme disease may probably also be the most common such infection in the rest of the world, but the necessary statistics are lacking. There are interesting differences in the way the disease presents in different parts of the world. In the USA arthritides are numerically more important than they are in Europe, where neurological symptoms – meningitis, meningoencephalitis, cranial nerve paralyses and peripheral neuritis – are more apparent. These differences may be related to demonstrable differences in strains of *B. burgdorferi* isolated from patients and ticks in different parts of the world (Welsh et al., 1992). The organism is currently divided into four genospecies, three of which are pathogenic (Van Dam *et al.*, 1993), while the fourth, a Japanese isolate, appears not to be so. *B. burgdorferi sensu stricto* provides almost all North American isolates, which are frequently associated with an arthritic clinical picture, while in Europe *B. afzelii* and *B. garinii* are found in patients with dermatological or neurological symptoms, respectively. The predominant clinical manifestation is not determined solely by the infecting genospecies, however; the internal environment of the patient may influence the picture. Patients with HLA-DR2 and HLA-DR4 phenotypes are more likely to develop Lyme arthritis (Steere *et al.*, 1990); and because antibody to the flagellin of *B. burgdorferi* binds to human axons, autoimmunity may play a role in the pathogenesis of neurological symptoms (Sigal and Tatum, 1988).

Lyme disease came to notice in Connecticut because of a progressive alteration in the ecology of quite large parts of New England; and the most thorough ecological investigation of the condition has been made in New England. An increasing amount of previously cultivated land has been left to its own devices for many years, and forest has been returning. As the forest grew, increasing numbers of white-tailed deer began to move into the region in the 1940s, providing a growing population of large mammalian hosts for *I. dammini*, although they may not be the most important host of the tick.

The ticks of both the American and European species mate during their autumn feeding period when they parasitize large mammals such as deer, sheep, horses or cattle. There is also evidence that dogs may not only carry ticks home to their owners, but may also experience intermittent arthritis caused by infection with the spirochaetes. The results of the autumn mating – the tiny larvae – appear in the spring and feed for up to five days on small mammals – white-footed mice in the USA, voles and other small rodents in Europe. Transovarial infection of larvae has been described, but is rare. A larva may, however, become infected if it feeds on an infected mammalian host. Having fed, the larva drops to the ground and moults to the nymphal stage. In late spring or early summer the nymph attaches itself to a small rodent, or a rabbit, or even a bird, and feeds again – perhaps for as long as 7 days. During this feed, the nymph may infect the host; or, if the host is already infected, it may infect an uninfected nymph. Which host supplies the blood meal is largely a matter of chance; the nymph will as readily attach itself to a passing human being as to any other mammal or bird.

Steere has noted that 'The primary areas now affected by Lyme disease in the United States, Europe, and Asia are sites near the terminal moraine of the glaciers of 15 000 years ago' (Steere, 1994). The significance of this observation is unclear. It may relate to the geography of the evolution of Ixodid ticks; but this throws no light on the reported occurrence of Lyme disease in Southern Africa and Australia. What looks like the worldwide distribution of *B. burgdorferi* may have resulted from the catholic choice of blood meal providers by the ticks, which includes birds. This could have led to infected nymphs being carried elsewhere by migratory birds.

The reservoir of spirochaetes is maintained in small mammals – probably rodents – thus permitting infection of the next crop of larvae. After the second blood meal the nymph returns to the undergrowth or other suitable habitat where the humidity is high and the temperature is above 7°C, and matures into an adult tick, ready for its third meal and mating in the autumn.

Within a few days (or sometimes weeks) of the infection by tick bite the patient develops a rash which increases rapidly in size – the erythema migrans. This often appears to start at the site of the tick bite, and is accompanied in perhaps half of the patients by secondary skin lesions on other parts of the body. Patients may also feel ill and tired, and develop headache, fever, muscle and joint pains, stiff neck, and lymphadenopathy. All the symptoms do not necessarily appear in every patient. Up to one patient in ten may have abdominal pain and vomiting, and if the history of tick bite is not known to the medical attendants the patient may be misdiagnosed as having an acute abdominal condition needing emergency surgery. Some patients who have forgotten about a past tick bite may fall ill many weeks or even years later with diseases of the nervous system, heart, or joints. In fact, about one patient in 12 develops some sort of heart complaint – which may be serious – and almost two-thirds have arthritis which occurs months and sometimes years after the tick bite. Like syphilis, Lyme disease is the result of multisystem infection. It ought, therefore, to be included in the differential diagnosis whenever the suspicion arises that more than one system is implicated in the patient's condition. Serological tests for specific antibody to *B. burgdorferi* can be done to provide the physician with valuable information. Although early in the infection antibody responses are poor, in most patients tests will be positive by about 6 weeks after the onset of illness. Negative tests should therefore be repeated after a suitable interval.

Timely treatment with antibiotics usually cures the disease and eradicates the infection, but this depends on correct diagnosis which, in turn, depends on a high index of suspicion in the mind of the physician. Although cure under treatment occurs more rapidly early in the disease, all stages should be curable by adequate oral doses of tetracycline, amoxicillin, third-generation cephalosporins or erythromycin, continued for up to 30 days if necessary. When the nervous system is implicated, large doses of intravenous penicillin or cephalosporin are indicated. Children under the age of 12 are treated with penicillin because of the risk that tetracycline may damage developing bones and teeth.

Since Lyme disease is an emerging disease in many parts of the world, and its importance may not have been appreciated by all members of the medical profession, it would be a sensible precaution for people bitten by ticks to report the fact to their doctors. If they are subsequently taken ill, the doctor's suspicions should be rapidly aroused and the appropriate treatment instituted. An emerging disease is not necessarily a new disease. Indeed, *B. burgdorferi* causes quite an old disease; symptoms and clinical accounts suggest that it has been around for a long time. It follows that an emerging disease is one which has but recently been recognized, and knowledge of it is not yet widely dispersed.

# References

Benach, J.L., Bosler, E.M., Hanrahan, J.P. *et al.* (1983). Spirochaetes isolated from the blood of two patients with Lyme disease. *New England Journal of Medicine* **308**, 740–742.

Burgdorfer, W., Barbour, A.G., Hayes, S.F. *et al.* (1982). Lyme disease – a tick borne spitochaetosis? *Science* **216**, 1317–1319.

Davis, D.H.S. (1948). Sylvatic plague in South Africa: history of plague in man, 1919–43. *Annals of Tropical Medicine & Parasitology* **42**, 207–217.

Duma, R.J., Sonenshine, D.E., Bozeman, F.M. *et al.* (1981). Epidemic typhus in the United States associated with flying squirrels. *Journal of the American Medical Association* **245**, 2318–2323.

Goldin, D., Champion, R.H., Rook, A. and Roberts, S.O.B. (1978). Erythema chronicum migrans in Britain. *British Medical Journal* **ii**, 1087.

Morse, S.S. and Schluederberg, A. (1990). Emerging viruses: the evolution of viruses and viral diseases. *Journal of Infectious Diseases* **162**, 1–7.

O'Connell, S. (1993). Lyme disease: a review. *Communicable Disease Report Review* **3**, R111–R115.

Relman, D.A. (1995). Lyme disease. *Scientific American Science and Medicine* **2**, 14.

Shrewsbury, J.F.D. (1971). *A History of Bubonic Plague in the British Isles.* Cambridge University Press, London.

Sigal, L.H. and Tatum, A.H. (1988). Lyme disease patients' serum contains IgM antibodies that cross react with neuronal antigens. *Neurology* **38**, 1439–1442.

Steere, A.C. (1994). Lyme disease: a growing threat to urban populations. *Proceedings of the National Academy of Science of the USA* **91**, 2378–2383

Steere, A.C., Malawista, S.E., Snydeman, D. *et al.* (1977). Lyme arthritis: an epidemic of oligoarthritis in children and adults in three Connecticut communities. *Arthritis and Rheumatism* **20**, 7–17.

Steere, A.C., Broderick, T.F and Malawista, S.E. (1978). Erythema chronica migrans and Lyme arthritis. Epidemiologic evidence for a tick vector. *American Journal of Epidemiology* **108**, 312–321.

Steere, A.C., Dwyer, E. and Winchester, R. (1990). Association of chronic Lyme arthritis with HLA-DR4 and HLA-DR2 alleles. *New England Journal of Medicine* **323**, 219-223.

Steere, A.C., Taylor, E., McHugh, G.L. and Logigian, E.L. (1993). The overdiagnosis of Lyme disease. *Journal of the American Medical Association* **269**, 1812–1816.

Technical Advisory Committee (1995) *Nature Medicine* **1**, 1237–1239.

Twigg, G. (1984a). *The Black Death: A Biological Reappraisal*, pp. 164–166. Batsford, London.

Twigg, G. (1984b). *The Black Death: A Biological Reappraisal.* pp. 157–161. Batsford, London.

Van Dam, A.P., Kuiper, H., Vos, K. *et al.* (1993). Different genospecies of *B. burgdorferi* are associated with distinct clinical manifestations of Lyme borreliosis. *Clinical Infectious Diseases* **17**, 708–717.

Welsh, J., Pretzman, C., Postic, D. *et al.* (1992). Genomic fingerprinting by arbitrarily primed polymerase chain reaction resolves *Borrelia burgdoferi* into three distinct phyletic groups. *International Journal of Systematic Bacteriology* **42**, 370–377.

Zinsser, H. (1935). *Rats, Lice, and History.* George Routledge, London.

# Chapter 10

# Vector-borne virus infections

Most vector-borne virus infections are carried by mosquitoes, but some, of particular regional importance, are transmitted by ticks, some by sandflies, while others – such as yellow fever virus – have been shown experimentally, or been found in nature, to be capable of transmission by both mosquitoes and ticks (Germain *et al.*, 1979). Virtually all of these infections are zoonoses with their primary vertebrate reservoirs in wildlife. Some, which may not necessarily include humans in their patterns of circulation, have complex infective cycles implicating birds and terrestrial vertebrates – usually, but not exclusively, mammals. For dengue fever, an infection of increasing importance, maintenance of human disease by the four serological types of the virus appears to depend on a cycle between humans and mosquitoes. Although there is a jungle circulation of dengue viruses between mosquitoes and non-human primates, it seems to be unrelated to either endemic or epidemic dengue in human populations; and viruses isolated from monkeys in the jungle cycle have been shown, by molecular analysis, to be distinct from those causing human disease (Kerschner *et al.*, 1986).

Human involvement in zoonoses commonly results from the intrusion of humans into the habitats of wildlife species which may be existing in harmony with infecting viruses which cause immunizing but non-pathogenic infections. A prime example of this is African yellow fever which, in nature, is cycled between monkeys and mosquitoes without, apparently, causing any major harm to either. This is presumably the end result of an ancient association between the parties which has led to an ecological climax state. When humans encroach on the habitat, offering alternate sources of the blood meals which female mosquitoes need before oviposition, they are exposed to the risk of infection with a virus which they have not previously experienced. Infection, in this case, leads to disease. In climates suitable for breeding, and when the feeding habits of the vector mosquitoes correspond in time and place with the movements of the intrusive humans, and the virus they carry is sufficiently virulent, the ingredients are in place for an epidemic outbreak of yellow fever. In tropical Africa, the home of yellow fever, several species of *Aëdes* act as vectors in different parts of the extensive yellow-fever belt, although in urban agglomerations *A. aegypti* is commonly implicated.

## Yellow fever

Yellow fever first came to prominence in the days of the West African slave trade which was stimulated by the establishment of sugar cane plantations in the Caribbean islands. The disease appeared in epidemic form on the island of Guadeloupe in 1684, and spread rapidly from there to other islands and the mainland. Both the virus and the vector mosquitoes were transferred to the virgin environment of the Caribbean islands via the notorious Middle Passage – the voyage of the slave ships between West Africa and the Americas.

At the outset in the New World, the spread of yellow fever depended on an infection cycle confined to humans and the *A. aegypti* mosquitoes descended from those which had made the crossing in containers of fresh water carried on the slave ships. Originally a breeder in holes in tree trunks in the jungle, *A. aegypti* rapidly adapted to urban life and laid its eggs in still water which had collected in all manner of receptacles. However, it also ventured from the coastal settlements to the surrounding jungle, where it found howler monkeys, and other New World simians, which provided blood meals, became infected and – unlike African monkeys – died; but this was not before they had infected indigenous *Haemogogus* and *Sabethes* mosquitoes taking a blood meal before oviposition. Many Central and South American monkeys are susceptible to, and reservoirs of, yellow fever. Unlike most New World monkeys, however, capuchins of the genus *Cebus* do not die when infected, and act as a substantial reservoir of the virus.

Although yellow fever is rightly regarded as a tropical disease, it has not, throughout its recorded history, been confined strictly to the tropics. After the spread of infection from the Guadeloupe outbreak in the mid-seventeenth century, there were epidemics of yellow fever at different times in the rest of the century and, subsequently, in such distant places as New York and Boston, where infected mosquitoes were transported by ship. There were repeated epidemics in the eighteenth century, some of which, starting in West Africa, were carried by sea to the Caribbean and the Canary Islands. Early in the nineteenth century epidemic yellow fever occurred in Cadiz and Barcelona, and also spread northwards on the Atlantic coast of the USA as far as Boston. Later, in mid-nineteenth century, there were outbreaks in St Nazaire in France and Swansea in Wales. In the New World, epidemic outbreaks occurred not only in the Caribbean islands, but also on the adjacent mainland of Central America and the coast of the Gulf of Mexico. The disease was also carried as far north as New Hampshire, Maine and Nova Scotia. *A. aegypti* does not normally survive at higher latitudes than the 10°C winter (January) isotherm in the northern hemisphere. In the late eighteenth century, however, there was a carry over of yellow fever in New York, Boston and Philadelphia from one year to the next. The vector mosquitoes were able to survive the winter, though this was more probably because they adopted a sheltered, indoor habitat than that they adapted swiftly to the rigours of the climate. Outbreaks of yellow fever were not uncommon in the valley of the Mississippi river as far north as Memphis. Epidemics continued to occur in the nineteenth century, frequently encompassing much of the eastern USA, sometimes as far north as Massachusetts and New Hampshire. By 1900 the Atlantic and Pacific coastal regions of Central and South America were endemic for yellow fever.

In 1900 the US Yellow Fever Commission, headed by Walter Reed, investigated the transmission of the disease in Cuba. A local physician, Dr Carlos Finlay, believed that Aëdine mosquitoes were involved, and Reed and his colleagues tested this theory very thoroughly and found that *Aëdes aegypti* was the vector of the disease. In the course of their experiments, which included exposing themselves to the bites of potentially infective mosquitoes to determine the mode of spread, a member of the Commission, J. W. Lazear, died of yellow fever. Vigorous mosquito-control activity to deny breeding places to *A. aegypti* in Cuba showed that the disease could be controlled. The same method was applied in the Panama Canal Zone, thus allowing the construction of the canal to be completed in the absence of epidemic yellow fever. Its subsequent use elsewhere in the hemisphere led to the elimination of urban yellow fever from the Americas by 1934. However, jungle yellow fever remained. From time to time it sweeps through the arboreal monkeys of Central America and Amazonia, doing much damage to their populations, and occasionally infecting humans who live or work in the jungle. In 1947, the Pan American Health Organization began a campaign to eradicate *A. aegypti* from the western hemisphere. In the 25 years to 1972 much progress was made, but in the USA and several countries of the Caribbean region there was little enthusiasm for the programme, both because of the cost and the ultimate intractability of the project. The mosquito therefore steadily reinfested many of the South American countries from which it had apparently been eliminated.

Studies in Francophone West Africa in the 1970s by Cornet and his colleagues (Germain *et al.*, 1981) confirmed and extended the findings of earlier workers, in both East and West Africa, of the considerable ecological complexity of yellow fever (Haddow *et al.*, 1947; Mattingly, 1949) (and by extrapolation, of dengue fever, carried by several of the same mosquitoes). This is a function not only of the ecology of the several species of aëdine mosquitoes involved, and their feeding relationships with the monkeys they infect, or are infected by, but also of the viruses which they carry and disseminate. Not only are there demonstrable antigenic differences between African and American strains of yellow fever virus, but African strains have been classified by RNA studies into three different topotypes (Deubel *et al.*, 1986), each of which is found in a different region of the continent with no geographical overlap. Two of these topotypes are West African, and the third was found in equatorial Africa and Ethiopia. The genetic stability demonstrated within each topotype shows that epidemic outbreaks of yellow fever are caused by spread of local viruses, and not by introductions of viruses from distant sources. Despite this, however, the standard 17D yellow-fever vaccine effectively immunizes against the disease in all parts of the world. The effectiveness of vaccination in the control of epidemic yellow fever in human populations has been clearly demonstrated by the history of the disease in West Africa where community vaccination was the norm in countries under French administration, but not in those governed by the British (Monath, 1991). The French colonial territories had far fewer yellow-fever epidemics than the British colonies, although the sylvatic cycle of infection between monkeys and mosquitoes was active under both jurisdictions. The lack of a vaccination policy in Anglophone Africa was not due either to stupidity or any sinister motive. Before the 17D strain of vaccine virus was developed, the French used a neurotropic strain of virus which was applied by scarification. The British believed the vaccine carried too great a risk of encephalitic complications, and refused to use it.

Since the end of the Second World War, and especially in the period since 1970, the urban population of Central and South America has increased hugely – partly by the influx of rural people seeking work and a better life in the towns, and largely by unrestrained child bearing, much of it the result of religious condemnation of artificial contraception. The overwhelming majority of these recruits to urban living exist in wretched poverty in periurban slums lacking such basic urban services as piped water supplies, sewage reticulations and garbage collection. The result is a high incidence of disease – especially gastrointestinal infections – and, because of the need to store water from stand pipes and other sources for cooking and cleaning, and because of the large, uncleared collections of bottles, jars, cans, discarded tyres and other objects capable of holding rainwater, there has been a huge increase in the size of *A. aegypti* populations.

This mosquito has not only once more become a scourge, or a potential scourge, in the western hemisphere, but its original range is being regained, and even expanded, in much of the rest of the world. It is improbable that this will mean a return to widespread epidemic outbreaks of yellow fever such as occurred in North America and Europe in the nineteenth century. The disease is so obvious, and would cause so many deaths, that even the most lackadaisical government would be forced to do something about it. In economically advanced countries this would mean not only a crash programme of mosquito elimination, but also extensive use of yellow-fever vaccine; though this could well be in short supply unless foresight had caused an emergency supply to be stock-piled. The countries with endemic yellow fever at present would no doubt be objects of sympathy were the disease to become epidemic, but a western world worrying about its own difficulties would probably offer little concrete help.

The existence of an environment suitable for a particular infection to flourish does not necessarily mean that it will flourish. In East Africa, for example, there is a continuous corridor, extending from Kenya and Tanzania, through Mozambique to the Eastern Transvaal and KwaZulu-Natal in the Republic of South Africa, which is inhabited by permanent populations of aëdine mosquitoes (including *A. aegypti*) and vervet monkeys (*Cercopithecus aethiops*), the basic elements in the epizootiology and epidemiology of yellow fever. Nevertheless, neither yellow-fever virus nor antibodies to it have ever been reported from the subtropical regions of the Republic, which have a suitable climate and an appropriate fauna for the support of a reservoir of the infection.

Much of India and South East Asia also have apparently suitable environments for the establishment of enzootic yellow fever. Despite what must be centuries of sea-borne commerce between East Africa and the west coast of India, largely in Arab dhows carrying breeding populations of *A. aegypti* in their stored water, if yellow-fever virus was ever transported across the Arabian Sea to India, it never took root. This may be because infection by other flaviviruses stimulates the production of sufficient concentrations of antibody against group structural antigens to protect against yellow-fever virus. However, there is no firm explanation of the continued freedom from yellow fever of such a large and heavily populated part of the world as South East Asia, despite the presence of aëdine mosquitoes – especially *A. aegypti*, local strains of which have been shown experimentally to be efficient vectors of the virus (Gillett and Ross, 1955).

Global warming, however, could induce such environmental changes in temperate climate zones as to make them suitable for the overwintering of tropical species of mosquitoes. The best estimate of the Working Group on Scientific Assessment of Climate Change of the Inter governmental Panel on Climate Change (IPCC) (1992) was that by the year 2050 global mean temperature will have increased by 1.5°C. The subsequent 1994 Report of the Scientific Assessment Working Group of IPCC (1994), on the whole, confirmed the earlier statement and made several projections of future trends, taking into account different rates of emission of $CO_2$ over periods of many years before stable concentrations of the gas are achieved. The 1995 projections of IPCC (Houghton *et al.*, 1995) confirm and extend the previous findings.

If the projections are reasonably accurate, a considerably increased area of the northern hemisphere landmass could become climatically suitable for the survival of numbers of what are, at present, tropical and subtropical arthropod vectors of several severe diseases with epidemic potential. With the demonstrated natural transovarial (or vertical) transmission of yellow-fever virus in mosquitoes (Haddow *et al.*, 1947), the complex ecological relationships between mosquitoes, monkeys and the virus could be greatly simplified to a relationship between vertically infected mosquitoes and humans. Should there be a permanent introduction of yellow fever into Europe or North America – which is not very likely – it could be efficiently controlled by preventive vaccination. More disturbing in the absence of effective vaccines would be the introduction of protozoal infections such as leishmaniasis or the re-introduction of malaria.

## Dengue fever

Another, and perhaps more imminent, hazard in those regions recently infested or reinfested by *A. aegypti* is the possible introduction of dengue fever to areas of the world at present free of it, and its reintroduction to regions from which it disappeared during the, eventually abortive, attempt to eradicate the vector from the western hemisphere during the period 1947 to 1972. In the late 1920s the range of *A. aegypti* was probably as great as it has ever been. Virtually the whole of subsaharan Africa, except for most of the Cape Province of the then Union of South Africa and about two-thirds of South-West Africa (now Namibia), was home to the insect. It was also present in the Nile Valley and most of the Mediterranean coast of the Maghreb, with an extension from Morocco to the southernmost tip of Spain. Turkey, part of the Russian Black Sea coast, Greece and the southern Balkan states, Sicily, the foot of Italy, the Ligurian coastal region and France's Mediterranean coastal region were also involved. The mosquito has been banished from these parts of Europe and near-to-Europe, which are climatically suitable for it; and it is to these parts that it is most likely to return if suitable breeding places are allowed to develop. In the Americas the mosquito has regained much – but not yet all – of its earlier range. The Indian subcontinent, South East Asia, Indonesia, the Philippines and Papua New Guinea are infested as heavily as ever they were, but the Australian range of the mosquito is now confined to the northern part of Queensland. Global warming may be expected to induce changes in the distribution of the mosquito.

The forecasting of future temperatures is complicated and difficult; there is always a range in the predictions, often a large range. Nevertheless, a mathematical model illustrated in the 1995 report of the IPCC (Houghton *et al.*, 1995) suggests that between 1880 and *c.* 2050 winter temperatures in the northern hemisphere may show an average increase of between 1 and 4°C, and in the southern hemisphere increases of up to 3°C. In Europe and North America this would indicate a probably significant shift northwards of the 10°C winter isotherm and a shift southwards in the southern hemisphere. It is impossible at this stage to be precise, but in both hemispheres the range of *A. aegypti* could be significantly increased. If dengue viruses are either introduced or spread naturally from their present areas of endemicity, there would be a considerable increase in the size of the human population that would be at risk of epidemic outbreaks of dengue fever.

Although the major vector of dengue fever is *A. aegypti* it can also be carried by *A. albopictus*, an Asian species which was found in Houston, Texas in 1985 and in Rio de Janeiro in 1986. These were separate importations which reached the Americas in used truck tyres which were to be recapped with new treads. Collections of these tyres were stored in the open in different parts of Asia before shipment to the recapping plants. During the storage period rainwater collected in them which was used by *A. albopictus* for oviposition. According to Monath (1994) about a fifth of the more than a million tyres a year being imported into the USA from Asia were unsuitable for recapping and were simply dumped, allowing the mosquito larvae they contained to mature into adult mosquitoes. Since then this species, which is described as winter hardy, has spread throughout the eastern USA, where it has every chance of naturalizing itself – even without global warming – unlike *A. aegypti* whose range is bounded, both north and south, by the 10°C winter isotherm.

Since the last quarter of the eighteenth century there have been at least ten pandemic outbreaks of dengue fever. The world may well expect more if the IPCC predictions turn out to be reasonably correct. Despite the spraying of aircraft interiors with insecticides after take-off from tropical airports and before landing in temperate-climate countries, the possibility exists that an aeroplane travelling from Africa or South East Asia could still deliver adult mosquitoes to a European environment in which they could breed.

Dengue fever is an acute febrile condition caused by infection with any of the four recognized serotypes of the dengue virus. The high fever lasts for up to a week, and is accompanied by severe pains in limbs and joints, which gave the disease the name of break-bone fever. Receptive female mosquitoes feeding on a patient within the viraemic phase of the illness – the first 2 or 3 days – become infected, but transmission to a susceptible subject cannot occur before the end of the extrinsic incubation period of 8–10 days. This is required for replication and dissemination of the virus within the insect, which allows it to reach the salivary glands and be present in the saliva when the infected female takes the next blood meal. The mosquito may remain infective for as long as 6 months.

During the Second World War outbreaks of dengue fever occurred in East Africa and innumerable military establishments in and around the Indian and Pacific Oceans. The movement of military personnel spread all four serotypes of the virus, and the movement of military *matériel* spread the vector mosquito very widely; but the disease remained virtually non-fatal. In 1950, however, there were deaths from dengue infection among children in Manila. The disease was characterized clinically by haemorrhagic phenomena (Dengue Haemorrhagic Fever – DHF) and, in the most severe cases, shock, which earned it the name of Dengue Shock Syndrome (DSS). DHF and the shock syndrome are manifestations of different degrees of severity of the same basic condition. Age and gender are risk factors. Children are at hazard more than adults, and girls more than boys. Despite dengue infection rates showing no difference by gender or age in the population at large, twice as many girls as boys between the ages of 4 and 14 years tend to be hospitalized with DHF/DSS.

After the Manila outbreak, DHF/DSS occurred in other countries of South East Asia and the Pacific rim. These were facilitated by the increased urbanization after the war, which was responsible for the growth of periurban slums without basic services, similar to what was happening in Central and South America at the same time. The need to store water for domestic purposes, and the lack of garbage collection, with all kinds of receptacles holding water, enriched the environment in which aëdine mosquitoes could (and did) breed – but, clearly, degraded the human environment. The presence of very large populations of mosquitoes and the several serotypes of dengue virus changed the pattern of dengue disease in South East Asia.

Investigations, in which Stuart Halstead (1988) was prominent, led to a clearer understanding of the condition. The overwhelming number of cases occurred in those subjected to a second, but not a third or fourth, infection with a serotype different from that which had caused the original attack of dengue. Antibody against the first infecting serotype combines with, but cannot neutralize, the newly infecting virus. The resulting complexes of antibody + antigen activate the classical pathway of complement and induce increased vascular permeability and some dysfunction of haemostasis which is accompanied by internal bleeding (DHF) which may proceed to shock (DSS), with case fatality rates of 2–10%.

Ethnicity appears to play some part in the pathogenesis of DHF/DSS. When the condition occurred in Cuba in 1981, there were disproportionately few black and mulatto children affected. According to Halstead, it does not occur in black Africans or in predominantly black populations of Caribbean islands.

In view of the ease with which both *A. aegypti* and *A. albopictus* seem to colonize suitable habitats and become naturalized in them, the environmental changes which may be expected in southern European countries as a result of global warming represent a potentially serious hazard to the public health of those countries. The influx of migrants from Africa is likely to increase as conditions in that continent continue to deteriorate. Some of the migrants may carry dengue viruses in their blood, which may be taken up by feeding female mosquitoes. This is not a risk which can be quantified, but experience in South East Asia, Central and South America, and the southern USA, suggests that it should not be hastily discounted by those responsible for guarding the public health. Control of dengue by eradication of the arthropod vector is improbable, if the recent history of attempts at worldwide control of *A. aegypti* is a reliable indicator. In any event, control of dengue must now include prevention of DHF/DSS, and this will require immunization of populations at risk by vaccines containing all four of the serotypes, possibly in the form of live, attenuated viruses, or perhaps as preparations of structural proteins. Dengue vaccine research is an active field.

## Japanese encephalitis

Japanese encephalitis is widely endemic in South East Asia, occurring in much the same area as dengue. Japanese encephalitis, like yellow fever and dengue, is caused by a flavivirus and, like them, offers excellent examples of the influence of environment on infection and epidemiology. Like other flaviviruses, the virus of Japanese encephalitis is mosquito borne. In their study of Japanese encephalitis in Sarawak, Simpson and his colleagues isolated the virus from several members of the genus *Culex,* and also from *Mansonia* spp. and *Anopheles* spp. (Simpson *et al.*, 1970). *Mansonia* mosquitoes are known to be receptive of the virus and to pass it to a variety of mammalian and avian hosts when females take their preovulatory blood meals. *Culex tritaeniorhynchus*, which feeds preferentially on pigs, but also bites humans, was the main vector for humans in a village environment, but *Culex gelidus* was virtually the only mosquito from which virus was isolated, at a distant piggery. The village had extensive adjacent rice fields, but very few pigs, while there were hundreds of pigs in the piggery, with almost no rice. Although there was a heavy incidence of infection in piggery pigs, the presence of never more than nine pigs in the village being studied indicated that these animals could not be the reservoir of the infections found by antibody studies in the villagers. Sixty-three per cent of 268 subjects tested had circulating neutralizing antibody to Japanese encephalitis virus.

In Japan, the most significant vertebrate maintenance hosts were water birds, particularly herons and egrets. Domestic pigs acted as amplifying hosts and *C. tritaeniorhynchus* fed on them. Being closely peridomestic in the summer, these mosquitoes increased the risk of human infections (Buescher and Scherer, 1959). In the Dyak village the inhabitants were indoors at the time of the greatest activity of the mosquitoes, which seldom bite indoors (Simpson *et al.*, 1974). Searching for other possible reservoirs of the infection, Simpson *et al.* tested sera from a variety of animals for antibody to the virus. Sixteen of 19 dogs were positive (84%), 19% of ducks, 18% of birds, especially waterhens and bitterns found in the paddy-fields, and 2% of bats, but no other animals. It appears that in Sarawak pigs act as amplifying hosts for the virus following a major increase in the population of *C. tritaeniorhynchus* (Simpson *et al.*, 1976). The increase in numbers of this species is closely associated with the routines of rice cultivation in Sarawak and reaches its greatest extent following very active breeding immediately before rice planting, when the fields would already be flooded. The dense population of mosquitoes attracts birds, which may bring the infection with them, or be infected after their arrival. The people working in the paddy-fields are exposed to the risk of infective bites by the mosquitoes, and the cycle of infection continues.

In a Sri Lankan study (Peiris *et al.*, 1993) mosquitoes were trapped, speciated and counted in six different areas of the island. From five of the areas sera were taken from humans, cattle, goats, pigs, dogs, domestic fowl, ducks, rabbits and sheep. In the sixth area only human beings, cattle, goats and pigs were sampled. Relevant culicine mosquitoes and serological indications of infection by Japanese encephalitis virus were sparse or lacking in stations at altitudes greater than 1200 metres, irrespective of rainfall and other climatic features which might be thought suitable for the multiplication of mosquitoes. The greatest incidence of antibody to the encephalitis virus in humans was found in low-lying country with rice as the main crop. Seroconversion in pigs, cattle, and goats followed a similar geographical pattern. Unlike the situation in Sarawak (Simpson *et al.*, 1970), the incidence of antibody in cattle and goats was a better predictor of the risk of human infection in areas where pigs were infected over a period of many months; but where the pigs were infected synchronously in relation to the monsoon rains, their infection was correlated with seroconversion in human beings.

Clearly, differences in both physical and socioeconomic environments influence the epidemic picture, as described with measles in Chapter 3. The inclusion of reservoir hosts and insect vectors introduces considerable complication into the epidemiology of any infectious disease. Indeed, the complexity is such that the epidemiology of yellow fever, Japanese encephalitis, or any other disease dependent on vectors and maintenance reservoirs of infection cannot be assumed to be the same in different environments. Even though the clinical appearance of the disease is similar in different settings, prevention depends on a thorough understanding of its epidemiology and this must be studied in each different setting.

An outbreak of Japanese encephalitis in Kerala caused 25 (or, according to some, 44) deaths (*Lancet*, 1996). Most of the dead were adults and, unusually, the outbreak occurred in the second, not the first, harvesting season for rice. It may be significant that pig breeding was introduced to the affected area in the previous year, but this opinion has been contested by members of the Indian research establishment. Another view is that a dam being built on the Varmada river may be associated with the outbreak – possibly by an increase in the available water surface attracting large numbers of birds including species known to be implicated in the ecology of Japanese encephalitis virus – and may well contribute to the spread of the infection in future. The ecological interactions in the disease situation clearly need to be established by careful investigation before the epidemiology of Japanese encephalitis in Kerala can be properly understood.

# References

Buescher, E.L. and Scherer, W.F. (1959). Ecological studies of Japanese encephalitis in Japan. IX: Epidemiological correlations and conclusions. *American Journal of Tropical Medicine and Hygiene* **8**, 719–722.

Deubel, V., Digoutte, J.P., Monath, T.P. and Girard, M. (1986). Genetic heterogeneity of yellow fever virus strains from Africa and the Americas. *Journal of General Virology* **67**, 209–213.

Germain, M., Saluzzo, J.F., Cornet, M. *et al.* (1979). Isolement du virus fièvre jaune a partir de Ia ponte et de larves d'une tique *Amblyomma variagatum*. *Comptes Rendus de l'Académie des Sciences [D] (Paris)* **289**, 635–637.

Germain, M., Cornet, M., Mouchet, J. *et al.* (1981). La fièvre jaune en Afrique: donnes recentes et conceptions actuelles. *Médicine Tropicale* **41**, 31–43.

Gillett, J.D. and Ross, R.W. (1955). The laboratory transmission of yellow fever by Malayan *Aëdes aegypti*. *Annals of Tropical Medicine and Parasitology* **49**, 63–65.

Haddow, A.J., Gillett, J.D. and Highton, R.B. (1947). The mosquitoes of Bwamba County, Uganda. V. The vertical distribution and biting-cycle of mosquitoes in rain-forest, with further observations on microclimate. *Bulletin of Entomological Research* **37**, 301–330.

Halstead, S.B. (1988). Pathogenesis of Dengue: challenges to molecular biology. *Science* **239**, 476–481.

Houghton, J.T., Meirofilho, L.G., Callander, B.A. *et al.* (eds) (1995). *Climate Change 1995. The Science of Climate Change*, Contribution of Work Group 1 for IPCC. Cambridge University Press, Cambridge.

Intergovernmental Panel on Climate Change (1992). Supplement: Scientific assessment of climate change.

Kerschner, J.A., Vorndam, A.V., Monath, T.P. and Trent, D.W. (1986). Genetic and epidemiological studies of dengue type 2 viruses by hybridization using synthetic deoxyoligonucleotides as probes. *Journal of General Virology* **67**, 2645–2661.

*Lancet* (1996). **347**, 678.

Mattingly, P.F. (1949). Studies on West African forest mosquitoes. Part 1. The seasonal distribution and biting cycle and vertical distribution of four of the principal species. *Bulletin of Entomological Research* **40**, 149–168.

Monath, T.P. (1991). Yellow fever: *Victor, Victoria?* Conqueror, conquest? Epidemics and research in the last forty years and prospects for the future. *American Journal of Tropical Medicine and Hygiene* **45**, 1–43.

Monath, T.P. (1994). Dengue: the risk to developed and developing countries. *Proceedings of the National Academy of Science of the USA* **91**, 2395–2400.

Peiris, J.S.M., Amerasinghe, F.P., Arunagiri, C.K. *et al.* (1993). Japanese encephalitis in Sri Lanka: comparison of vector and virus ecology in different agro-climatic areas. *Transactions of the Royal Society of Tropical Medicine and Hygiene* **87**, 541–548.

Report of the Scientific Assessment Working Group of IPCC (1994). Radiative Forcing of Climate Change.

Simpson, D.I.H., Bowen, E.T.W., Way, H. J. *et al.* (1974). Arbovirus infections in Sarawak, October 1968–February 1970: Japanese encephalitis virus isolations from mosquitoes. *Annals of Tropical Medicine and Parasitology* **68**, 393–404.

Simpson, D.I.H., Bowen, E.T.W., Platt, G.S. *et al.* (1970). Japanese encephalitis in Sarawak: virus isolation and serology in a Land Dyak village. *Transactions of the Royal Society of Tropical Medicine and Hygiene* **64**, 503–510.

Simpson, D.I.H. Smith, C.E.G., Marshall, T.F. de C. *et al.* (1976). Arbovirus infections in Sarawak: the role of the domestic pig. *Transactions of the Royal Society of Tropical Medicine and Hygiene* **70**, 66–72.

# Chapter 11

# Protozoal infections

## Malaria

Human beings are liable to get malaria when they share the environment with flourishing populations of vector mosquitoes infected with the causal parasites. This means, today, that malaria is a disease of the tropics and subtropics. It was not always so. Within living memory malaria was an indigenous disease widely present in regions of temperate climate including Europe where, in its heyday, it was active as far north as Finland, where the last transmissions occurred in 1948 (Bruce-Chwatt and Zulueta, 1980). In Central and Eastern Europe malaria was present into the 1960s, when it disappeared, partly because of a general improvement in environmental standards in the post-war period, and partly because of campaigns to eradicate mosquitoes – based largely upon the use of residual spraying of dwellings with persistent insecticides, especially DDT. In former Yugoslavia, for example, the last indigenous cases of falciparum malaria were reported in 1947, and vivax malaria in 1964 (Bruce-Chwatt and Zulueta, 1980).

Malaria tends to be absent at altitudes above 2000 metres because at this elevation the environment is generally unsuitable for the breeding of mosquitoes. This may not hold, however, if global warming makes climates at these altitudes more congenial for the insects.

After Ross showed in 1897 that the infection was spread by the bites of infected female mosquitoes of the genus *Anopheles*, environmental and social improvements were accompanied by reductions both in anopheline populations and the incidence of malaria in many European countries. By the middle of the twentieth century the main foci of European malaria were in the warmer, southern parts of the continent and the Mediterranean and Aegean islands. It was also still present in Britain and the Netherlands. In Britain, the last reported case of indigenous malaria occurred in Lancashire, in 1957 (Shute, 1963). In the Netherlands, more than 15 000 indigenous cases were reported in 1946, largely due to the breakdown of control measures during the Second World War.

Reports dwindled to single figures by 1956, and to zero by 1962. In much of Europe the vectors were members of the *An. maculipennis* complex, represented in Britain and the Netherlands mainly by *An. atroparvus*, which breeds preferentially in brackish water.

Both the mosquitoes and the parasites they carry have complex life cycles. The mosquito lays its eggs either in or very close to water. A larva develops (usually within a few days, depending upon the ambient temperature), and lives and feeds in the water, suspended under the surface by special structures, and takes in oxygen through spiracles at the surface of the water. As the larva grows it moults three times and in the final moult the fourth larval instar becomes a pupa, which develops into the adult – no longer aquatic, but a terrestrial and aerial insect. According to Bruce-Chwatt (1980), of the approximately 400 known species of *Anopheles*, 'only about 60 are important vectors of malaria under natural conditions'.

Human malaria is caused by four species of protozoal parasite: *Plasmodium falciparum, P. malariae, P. ovale* and *P. vivax*. Part of their development – the extrinsic cycle – happens in the mosquito vector, and part – the intrinsic cycle – in the infected human host. A female mosquito must take a blood meal before oviposition. If infected when she does so, she injects into the host, with her saliva, *sporozoites* which circulate briefly in the blood before those that are not destroyed by phagocytes enter liver cells, where they divide repeatedly into several thousand *merozoites*. This, the pre-erythrocytic phase, lasts from 5 to 16 days, depending on the species. At the end of this period infected liver cells break open and the merozoites enter the blood stream where they invade red cells and undergo asexual division to produce *schizonts*. When fully mature the schizonts produce more merozoites which, when the red cells rupture, are released into the circulation and infect fresh red cells. This process continues until the subject either dies or develops sufficient immunity to hold it in check. In vivax, ovale and falciparum malaria the freeing of new crops of merozoites occurs after 48 hours, accompanied by fever and rigors, and in malariae infection, after 72 hours. After several production cycles some of the merozoites are differentiated sexually into male and female *gametocytes* which invade red cells, where they grow, but do not divide.

When a female *Anopheles* takes a meal of human blood containing malaria parasites, the merozoites and the red cells are digested, but the gametocytes develop further. The female gametocyte matures into a *macrogamete*, while the nucleus of the male gametocyte divides into four or eight *flagella* which break free from the originating cell as *microgametes*. In the mosquito's stomach macrogametes are fertilized by microgametes with the formation of zygotes which develop into elongated *oökinetes*, and then *oöcysts*. The nuclei of the oöcysts divide frequently to form numerous spindle-shaped *sporozoites* which are freed into the coelome of the mosquito, from where large numbers of them reach the salivary glands. The mosquito is now armed and infective, and remains so for the rest of her life. When she takes a blood meal sporozoites are injected with her saliva and enter the blood stream of the host, and the cycle of malarial infection is initiated once more. The extrinsic cycle is temperature dependent. Below 15°C *P. vivax* does not develop. The sexual cycle takes 16 days at 20°C and 8–10 days at 28°C. The sexual cycle in *P. falciparum* takes 22 days at 20°C, and 10 or 11 days at 25–28°C. Vivax malaria could thus occur in many parts of the world, given that the vectors are able to establish themselves, but rapid reproduction and circulation of *P. falciparum* would be more likely to be successful in consistently warm and humid climates.

When Ross elucidated the role of mosquitoes in the natural history of malaria, many thought that the epidemiology of the disease, and with it control measures, would unfold seamlessly. But because there are four different parasites and many different species of mosquito involved in widely disparate parts of the world, the epidemiology of malaria is neither simple nor all inclusive: it must be studied closely in each of the settings around the world in which the disease occurs if it is to be sufficiently well understood to guide the necessary preventive measures; and preventive measures are very necessary. Worldwide morbidity from malaria is not known with any precision, but there may be about 200 million cases a year, with between two and three million deaths.

The greatest number of malarial deaths is probably in subsaharan Africa, where *P. falciparum* occurs commonly, carried mainly by *An. gambiae* and *An. funestus*, both of which feed preferentially on human blood. The likelihood that parasites will be transmitted from vector to human host, and complete their intrinsic life cycle, depends on the population density, feeding habits and longevity of the mosquitoes. Both *An. gambiae* and *An. funestus* feed frequently and are (for mosquitoes) long lived. This is important because a mosquito must feed on human blood twice to be able to transmit malaria. In the first feed it acquires gametocytes and is infective only after completion of the extrinsic cycle, which may take 10 days or more, depending on the ambient temperature, and as many as 25% of the females in a population may die each day.

In parts of West Africa and much of central Equatorial Africa malaria is holoendemic, which is to say that there is considerable transmission of parasites throughout the year and a high level of immunity, especially in adults. It follows that young children are the most heavily affected sector of the population and, where *P. falciparum* is the most frequent parasite, the one suffering the highest mortality. This is particularly likely in those parts of the continent where *An. gambiae* is the most important vector of malaria, since much of the disease incidence results from human activity. This mosquito is frequently found in puddles of water open to the direct heat of the tropical sun – puddles which form in shallow depressions caused by cultivation or claypits, or by human or animal footprints. Any such collection of water is suitable, including that in earthwalled containers, but not – unlike many aëdine mosquitoes – in containers such as empty tin cans or discarded tyres. According to J.D. Gillett (1971), 'It is often hard to find the species round the shores of the great lakes until they have been disturbed or developed by man ... Introduce man, and *An. gambiae* follows within a month.' The other major African vector, *An. funestus*, lays its eggs in clear, clean water, often at the edges of fast running streams where they are sheltered by weeds. Both of these mosquitoes feed in increasing numbers from dusk until dawn. In warm weather enormous numbers of *An. gambiae* may appear a few days after rain. Fresh out of the pupa, the insects are not infected, but when feeding, some of the females may take, with the blood, gametocytes which enter and complete the extrinsic cycle. The cycle of infection has been initiated, and the mosquito will remain infective for the rest of its life. A high level of endemicity, and hence of immunity, precludes epidemic outbreaks of malaria, and in these circumstances the disease is described as stable.

The plasmodia acquire their metabolites both from the haemo-globin of the red cells which they parasitize and from substances in the plasma. Infection by *P. falciparum* causes the most severe form of malaria, possibly because – unlike the other plasmodia – it infects red cells of all ages, while *P. vivax* and *P. ovale* prefer reticulocytes and *P. malariae* prefers mature red cells. Falciparum malaria is therefore characterized by a greater degree of parasit-aemia and greater morbidity and mortality than is found in disease caused by the other species. Malaria in general causes fever, anaemia and reduced perfusion of tissues. When there is a high parasitaemia there may be severe haemolysis with haemoglobin-uria – so-called blackwater fever – and renal failure. An important complication of falciparum infection is cerebral malaria – a result of the red cells becoming stiffer and stickier, and thus liable to block cerebral capillaries.

In the African – holoendemic – situation, most people, including infants and young children, receive several infective bites each year, but by about the age of 5 the survivors have developed sufficient immunity to keep the infection and disease under a useful degree of control. With such a high degree of endemicity, epidemic outbreaks of malaria do not occur. Those with no experience of malaria, however, such as tourists from Europe or North America, are very much at risk if they do not regularly take suitable antimalarial drugs (if they are available for the strains of parasite circulating in that locality), and adopt sensible mosquito-avoidance practices.

In other regions, such as Sri Lanka, parts of India and South America, transmission of parasites fluctuates from year to year and there is little immunity in the population. Under these conditions malaria is epidemiologically unstable and epidemic outbreaks are liable to occur, especially after heavy rains and warm weather have established a suitable environment for large-scale mosquito breeding. In India there are about two million cases a year, with about a third being falciparum malaria.

In continental Europe and parts of Britain, malaria was present for centuries in the unstable form. Although cases occurred in the appropriate part of the year, they were not necessarily numerous unless there was a flush of mosquitoes, when there might be epidemic outbreaks of the disease. Because the population was not regularly reinfected, unlike the situation in holoendemic areas, it lacked immunity, and the epidemics therefore tended to be widespread. The Romans apparently thought the Thames Valley was an unhealthy posting because of the fevers which afflicted their legions. In more recent centuries the fevers from which people suffered were known as the ague – a term used broadly to refer to a variety of conditions characterized by high fever, including typhus, among others. Although not all cases of ague were malaria, by the seventeenth century the intermittent fever described by Sydenham was, without much doubt, malaria; and from then on most (but still not all) ills described as ague were probably malaria.

The English regions most heavily affected seem to have been the salt-marsh areas of Kent and Essex, where *An. atroparvus* – a mosquito which lays its eggs in brackish water – was very common, and can still be found. The disease was not confined to Essex and Kent. Lambeth and Westminster were recognized as centres of the ague in London, and it was active in much of the country, where it may have been related not only to unhygienic environments and lack of drains, but also to pigs being kept in less than ideal conditions, close to human habitations. Mosquitoes found the warm, moist conditions of the pigsties congenial, and the pigs a ready source of blood meals. They were able to overwinter with the pigs, or even in the farmhouse kitchen, where they were content to feed on human blood, although – unlike *An. gambiae* – it was not their first choice. On the Isle of Grain before and soon after the First World War, thousands of *An. atroparvus* were present in pigsties throughout the year. Between 1917 and 1921 481 cases of malaria were reported in the inhabitants of the Isle, while between 1941 and 1948 there were only 38 cases. This was ascribed to the armed services not posting men returned from malarious parts of the world to the 'dangerous' parts of Kent and Essex, as had happened during and after the First World War. The last reported indigenous case of malaria in England occurred in Lancashire in 1957, apparently carried by *An. atroparvus* found in an unhygienic local pigsty. Two cases reported from Brixton in 1952 were thought to have been infected by *An. plumbeus*, a mosquito which breeds exclusively in tree holes containing water. It can be found all over England where there are suitable trees, and in laboratory experiments was an efficient carrier of both *P. vivax* and *P. falciparum* (Shute, 1963).

As global warming develops, those areas of Britain and Europe where anopheline mosquitoes still exist must be regarded as possible sites for appearance of foci of malaria. British and European malaria was caused by *Plasmodium vivax*. As noted above, this species cannot complete its extrinsic cycle at temperatures less than 15°C. Late spring, summer and early autumn temperatures in most of Britain and Europe could therefore comfortably support not only the likely vectors, but also this parasite if it were to be reintroduced. With the movement of people from South East Asia, where *P. vivax* is the predominant species, it is all too easy to envisage such a reintroduction – especially because one of the features of vivax malaria is the late occurrence of relapses in people diagnosed and apparently cured years earlier. In the liver-cell, or exoerythrocytic, stage of the intrinsic cycle, vivax parasites may persist – sometimes for years – as hypnozoites (analogous to the sort of secret agents, beloved of spy thrillers, known as 'sleepers') before regaining activity and precipitating a relapse (Krotoski *et al.*, 1982). The Intergovernmental Panel on Climate Change believes that by the year 2050 average global temperature will have increased by between 1°C and 2.5°C. This estimate is, of course, an approximate projection reached by the use of complex, and not certifiably complete, mathematical models. It is, nevertheless, the considered opinion of a large, international body of meteorologists (Reports of the Scientific Assessment Working Group of IPCC, 1994) which cannot be disregarded out of hand. Even at the lower end of the range of temperature increase that the Working Group offers, summer temperatures are bound to be significantly greater than the average – possibly high enough to support the extrinsic cycle of *P. falciparum*. Both *An. atroparvus* and *An. plumbeus* are able to sustain the extrinsic cycle of *P. falciparum*, and immigrants from Africa and other regions where this parasite is predominant could readily bring it with them.

Human interference in the environment will certainly cause changes in the local ecology, and very likely exert a more distant influence, too. Among the more potent changes instituted by mankind are alterations in water resources – dam building, and the introduction of irrigated agriculture, and so on. Rice cultivation, for example in the Camargue and southern Italy, which requires the flooding of fields in the earlier stages of the growing process, can be expected to promote the rapid multiplication of mosquitoes at discrete times of the year, with subsequent epidemic outbreaks in regions of unstable malaria. Unrestricted logging of tropical lowland rain forests may have a similar effect by exposing timber fellers working in the forest and people living and working on its fringes to jungle mosquitoes. This has happened both in Amazonia and South East Asia, where severe epidemic outbreaks of malaria have followed the meeting with efficient vectors among the jungle mosquitoes (Bradley, 1995). Where the forest has been clear-felled these mosquitoes can no longer breed, and the incidence of malaria declines; but this does not justify the destruction of tropical rain forests.

If, in conditions of global warming, malaria does return to countries and regions from which it has disappeared more or less spontaneously (i.e., without specific effort by public health authorities), or from which it has been eradicated by positive effort, it could well be a mistake to attack it *en masse* as in the eradication campaigns undertaken in the post-war years with the support of WHO. Some of these campaigns, as in Sardinia and the Balkan countries, were successful, but in other parts of the world, such as India, initial success in greatly reducing the incidence was followed by return of the disease. Today's goal is control (Bradley, 1991) through avoidance of exposure to potentially infective mosquitoes, and chemoprophylaxis and treatment of infection, together with sensible management of the environment aimed at minimizing the breeding of mosquitoes.

## Leishmaniasis

Infection by protozoal parasites of the genus *Leishmania* occurs in at least 88 countries – tropical, subtropical and temperate – around the world. Several species, *L. tropica* and *L. major* in particular, cause cutaneous lesions known as 'Oriental sore' in North Africa, the Middle East, the Indian subcontinent, and in a few foci in southern parts of Europe. These lesions eventually heal with scarring. In South America, cutaneous leishmaniasis is caused by *L. mexicana* and *L. braziliensis*. Although the lesions caused by *L. braziliensis*, like those of *L. mexicana,* heal, the parasite spreads from the site of infection and after a variable period, distant areas of skin and mucous membrane become the sites of persistent, destructive ulceration called *espundia*. Visceral leishmaniasis in temperate climate countries around the Mediterranean Sea is caused by *L. infantum* (which may also cause cutaneous lesions (Pozio *et al.*, 1985)). Kala azar, or visceral leishmaniasis caused by *L. donovani*, is found in the Indian subcontinent and parts of the Middle East. Most infections are subclinical, but if active and untreated, may ultimately be fatal. All *Leishmania* infections are spread by the bites of several species of sandfly, in which the parasites, extracellular and flagellated, are known as *promastigotes*. In mammalian hosts the *amastigote* parasite is intracellular and unflagellated. The leishmaniases are zoonotic. The *Leishmania* which cause cutaneous lesions have their animal reservoirs in various species of rodent, and the infections tend to be acquired in situations – often rural – where the vector has access to both rodent and human populations which do not necessarily have to be close to each other, since some species of sandfly can fly distances of at least 2 km (Killick-Kendrick *et al.*, 1988). The animal reservoirs of the *Leishmania* causing the visceral disease are dogs and other canids. Dogs are the most important reservoirs in Europe, while in North Africa and the Middle East, dogs provide urban and periurban reservoirs of infection, while foxes and jackals take this role additionally in rural environments.

In addition to the commonly recognized tropical and subtropical areas of leishmanial infection, there are European foci in France, Italy, Spain and Greece, as well as some Mediterranean islands. Among the best studied is a focus in the Cévennes in southern France, which has been investigated for many years by Professor J.-A. Rioux of the Faculté de Médecine of the University of Montpellier, and Professor R. Killick-Kendrick of Imperial College, London and their collaborators. Their studies show clearly how infection may be influenced by environment.

*Leishmania infantum* is the cause of canine leishmaniasis and human visceral leishmaniasis in the Cévennes. It is carried by the sandfly *Phlebotomus ariasi* which has been shown experimentally to transmit the visceral infection to dogs (Rioux *et al.*, 1980). Although the sandfly is found at altitudes higher than 1000 metres above sea level, human beings are at greatest risk of infection on the middle slopes of hillsides at altitudes between 300 and 500 metres, corresponding to the regions of greatest density of the fly (Rioux et al., 1980). Ambient temperature – also part of the physical environment – influences the incidence of visceral leishmaniasis. The condition is not seen at altitudes greater than 600 metres although, as noted above, P. ariasi is present at altitudes above 1000 metres. Female sandflies were caught at night and confined with a heavily infected dog. In the morning engorged females were separated and held at temperatures between 10 and 25°C, increasing temperature increased the overall proportion of infected flies, accelerated the multiplication of promastigotes in the midgut, controlled the migration of parasites anteriorly into the thoracic midgut, and promoted their attachment to the wall of the stomodaeal valve (Rioux et al., 1985), all of which increased the probability of the flies being infective when next they took a blood meal. The optimal temperature was 25°C. Temperatures of less than 5°C and more than 30°C killed the sandflies and, as a rule, the parasites. The temperature difference at 1000 metres or more, and the reduced density of the fly population at those altitudes, could well account for the cut off of infection above 600 metres.

The range of sandflies extends northwards to latitude 40°N (Lewis, 1973). The Channel Islands, where Phlebotomus perniciosus was identified in 1923 (Marett, 1923), the Isles of Scilly, and – on the Cornish mainland – the Lizard are within or close to this limit. This species is an established vector of L. infantum in France, Italy, Malta, Spain and parts of North Africa. If, by the year 2050, global warming has increased average surface temperature by 1.0 to 2.5°C, summer temperatures in southern England would allow phlebotomine sandflies to breed annually. As Professor R. Killick-Kendrick has pointed out in a personal communication: 'The winters in the UK would be no barrier to colonisation by sandflies because the Palearctic species of Phlebotomus overwinter as the 4th instar larvae'. He also says: 'the comparatively long incubation of the disease [visceral leishmaniasis] means that importation of infected dogs is not controlled by six months' quarantine. With slight changes in the weather, I see no reason why we should not expect transmission'.

The likelihood of leishmaniasis becoming a widespread health hazard may be remote, but it should be borne in mind because global warming may well be accompanied by the expansion of existing habitats suitable for sandflies and, hence, enlargement of rural foci of the infection. Increasing numbers of travellers between

Britain and Mediterranean Europe could lead to the importation of *Leishmania* species. Abolition of the rabies quarantine would presumably allow British dogs to accompany their owners to southern Europe where they could acquire leishmanial infection. If phlebotomine vectors find suitable environments to colonize in southern Britain, if not further north, there would be a reasonable likelihood of transfer of parasites to dogs and from dogs to foxes. Visceral leishmaniasis would then be established as a permanent and intractable disease in Britain.

The possibility that global warming may facilitate the introduction to temperate-climate regions of disease generally regarded as tropical ought to stimulate either national or regional authorities (or both) to construct surveillance mechanisms able to recognize early indications of the appearance of such conditions, and public-health structures able to react rapidly against them.

# References

Bradley, D.J. (1991). Malaria – whence and whither? In *Malaria: Waiting for the Vaccine* (G.A.T. Targett, ed.), pp. 12–29 John Wiley, Chichester.

Bradley, D.J. (1995). The epidemiology of malaria in the tropics and in travellers. In *Clinical Infectious Diseases* vol 2, *Malaria* (G. Pasvol, ed.), chap 1, Ballière Tindall, London.

Bruce-Chwatt, L.J. (1980). *Essential Malariology*. Heinemann Medical, London.

Bruce-Chwatt, L.J. and de Zulueta, J. (1980). *The Rise and Fall of Malaria in Europe*. Oxford University Press, Oxford.

Gillett, J.D. (1971). Mosquitoes p. 39. Weidenfeld & Nicolson, London.

Killick-Kendrick, R., Wilkes, T.J., Bailly, M. *et al.* (1986). Preliminary field observations on the flight speed of a phlebotomine sandfly. *Transactions of the Royal Society of Tropical Medicine and Hygiene* **80**, 138–142.

Krotoski, W.A., Collins, W.E., Bray, R.S. *et al.* (1982). Demonstration of hypnozoites in sporozoite-transmitted Plasmodium vivax infection. *American Journal of Tropical Medicine and Hygiene* **31**, 1291–1293.

Lewis D.J. (1973). Phlebotomidae and Psychodidae (sandflies and mothflies). In *Insects and other Arthropods of Medical Importance* (K.G.V. Smith, ed.), pp. 155–177. British Museum (Natural History), London.

Marett, P.J. (1923). A note on the capture of a *Phlebotomus perniciosus* ♂ in Jersey, C.I. *Transactions of the Royal Society of Tropical Medicine and Hygiene* **17**, 267.

Pozio, E., Gramiccia, L., Gradoni, L and Amerio, P. (1985). Isolation of the agent causing cutaneous leishmaniasis in Italy and its visceralization in inbred hamsters. *Transactions of the Royal Society of Tropical Medicine and Hygiene* **79**, 260–261.

Report of the Scientific Assessment Working Group of IPCC (1994). Radiative forcing of climate change.

Shute, P.G. (1963). Indigenous malaria in Britain since the First World War. *Lancet* **ii**, 576–578.

Rioux, J.-A., Killick-Kendrick, R., Leaney, A.J. *et al.* (1979). Écologie des Leishmanioses dans le sud de la France 11. La Leishmaniose viscérale canine: succès de la transmission expérimentale 'Chien → Phlébotome → Chien' par le piqûre de *Phlebotomus ariasi* Tonnoir, 1921. *Annales de Parasitologie* **54**, 401–407.

Rioux, J.-A., Killick-Kendrick, R., Perieres, J. *et al.* (1980) Écologie des Leishmanioses dans le Sud de la France 13. Les sites de 'flanc de coteau', biotopes de transmission privilégiés de la Leishmaniose viscérale en Cévennes. *Annales de Parasitologie* **55**, 445–453.

Rioux, J.-A., Aboulker, J.P., Lanotte, G. *et al.* (1985). Écologie de Leishmanioses dans le Sud de la France 21 – Influence de la température sur le développement de *Leishmania infantum* Nicolle, 1908 chez *Phlebotomus ariasi* Tonnoir, 1921. Étude expérimentale. *Annales de Parasitologie humaine et comparée* **60**, 221–229.

# Chapter 12

# A look into the future

Although the dream of a disease-free world is illusory, a few of the many infections which harry humanity may, perhaps, be consigned to share the oblivion of smallpox. Many epidemiologically important diseases can already be controlled by vaccination, although coverage of populations at risk is not uniformly wide enough. Thanks to the Expanded Programme of Immunization initiated by WHO, poliomyelitis is a diminishing threat, though a problem yet, in the developing world; but there are still too many cases of measles and rubella, even in industrially developed societies. The epidemic outbreaks of diphtheria in parts of the former USSR following administrative breakdown of public-health control, are a salutary example of the urgent need to maintain vaccination regimens consistently if such disasters are to be prevented. Some widespread diseases such as cholera, dysentery and other gastrointestinal infections, which are at present running free, may – in the near future – be controllable by regular and sustained application of new vaccines under development. In the long term, permanent control of these infections can only be guaranteed by the introduction of properly maintained, clean, piped water supplies and sewage reticulations, and regular, frequent clearance of garbage.

The immediate and long-term costs of such interventions are very high, however, and the countries which need them most are least able to afford them. These are the very countries whose rapid population growth makes it almost impossible for them to generate enough wealth to afford what, to their people, are almost unimaginable luxuries, but in the developed world are basic necessities. In the absence of the massive capital investment needed to install this sort of infrastructure, cheap, safe and effective vaccines would be the most cost-effective way of significantly reducing high incidences of disease. Inexpensive vaccines able to establish herd immunity against two of the major killing infections – tuberculosis and malaria – are sorely needed. When they are eventually available, their deployment will depend considerably on the solution of severe logistic problems. Some of the experience gained in the Smallpox Eradication Programme will certainly be applicable. Two of the advantages enjoyed by the Smallpox Programme were a vaccine which was applied percutaneously and not by syringe and needle, and a simple method – the scar survey – of determining the immunity of individuals and populations. Analogous methods for other infections would be invaluable. Single-dose oral vaccines and vaccines without a need for refrigeration would greatly improve the prospects of successful campaigns against many of the diseases which beset the world. The future, however, depends not only on improved health care and widely deployed preventive medicine, but also on solutions to the economic and social problems of, especially, the poorer countries of the world.

The agricultural and health sciences are not a little responsible for the present state of the world. Much has been done to reduce the impact of hunger and disease. Despite the frighteningly large number of infective deaths each year, a smaller proportion of the global population dies at a young age now than 50 years ago. Death control has been comparatively successful, and despite the wide presence of malnutrition, food production has improved in many countries to the point where famine, although relatively rare, is horrifying when it does occur, as in Ethiopia and the Southern Sudan in recent years. Thanks partly to forces which cause children to be regarded as economic assets, partly to religious bigotry, birth rates in many of the poorer parts of the world are still out of control, causing rapid increases in populations. Death control and agricultural improvement between them have removed the two most potent natural mechanisms limiting population growth. Humans themselves have become the most destructive biological agents which threaten the future.

Overcrowded habitats lead to overcultivation of farmlands, erosion of soils and loss of fertility, followed by migration in search of land for the production of food. All too often unsuitable areas such as tropical rain forests are destroyed in the attempt to establish a satisfactory life, compounding the destruction wrought by commercial overexploitation. There is little doubt that much of the destruction impinges on the global weather pattern. So, too, does increasing urbanization caused by rural overpopulation. The increasing industrialization of major Third World countries which accompanies and encourages urbanization is itself an important factor adding to the effects of radiative forcing of climate change,

The growth of populations, whether of bacteria or any other type of organism, can be seen to be limited – generally by the availability of nutrients. Humans seem to be an exception to this limitation of population size, despite the grim prediction by the Reverend Thomas Malthus in his *Essay on Population* in 1798. He believed that populations would collapse because their growth would outstrip the capacity of agriculture to feed them. For 200 years, however, agriculture has managed – sometimes more, sometimes less – to keep pace with the world's demand for food; but to claim, as agricultural experts do, that because agriculture has, in the past, kept pace, it will inevitably continue to do so, is logically untenable. Agriculture *may* continue successfully to feed the multitudes, but there can be no certainty about it. Improvements in agriculture which have been responsible for its success so far depend (as in other science-based activities) on advances in science and technology; but since these are unpredictable, a future depending upon them is also unpredictable. It follows, therefore, that if the conditions under which agriculture has operated for 200 years are severely altered, agricultural outcomes must be even more unpredictable.

This is clearly not a reason for abandoning death control; but if disease and hunger are to be controlled in any meaningful way, birth control must be promoted vigorously despite obscurantist religious views to the contrary. The bitter end predicted by Malthus has been repeatedly postponed, but with radiative forcing of climate change an established fact, it is possible to foresee a time when food production may no longer be expanded to meet the needs of relentlessly expanding population. Commercial overexploitation of natural resources, the accelerating overpopulation of the Earth, and the climatic changes expected to accompany global warming will have so degraded the human environment that it will no longer be able to support all of the teeming thousands of millions struggling to stay alive.

Global warming may already have caused severe climatic perturbations. Droughts in Russia, Australia, North Africa and parts of the USA were followed by greatly reduced cereal harvests in 1996, with world stocks of cereals at their lowest for 20 years. The poor harvest of 1996 may, of course, be a freak – but it may not. Repeated poor harvests because of climate change will do little to comfort the world's human population of 5700 million, estimated to reach 8300 million by 2025 – an increase of 45.6% in less than 30 years.

With a population change of this size, and probably worsening climatic conditions for agriculture in several important food-producing parts of the world, we may expect widespread malnutrition, increasing episodes of famine, and deteriorating hygiene.

These are all conditions which depress immunity, which in turn will allow latent tuberculosis to regain activity, with wide transmission of tubercle bacilli in affected populations. Drought, crop failure and famine will encourage people to aggregate in unhygienic circumstances very suitable for the transmission of epidemic typhus in those parts of the world where there is at present a small incidence of endemic louse-borne typhus.

New agents and new diseases have appeared and will continue to appear. Infection with HIV which leads in most, if not all, cases eventually to AIDS, is probably the major cause of death in subsaharan Africa; an estimated 75% of the world's cases of AIDS are in Africa. Because AIDS patients' immune systems are seriously impaired and they are mostly malnourished, they have virtually no resistance to many infections. Tuberculosis is particularly important because it is so widespread in Africa. An extraordinarily high proportion of the population of Africa is infected by the tubercle bacillus, and if they are not already suffering from open pulmonary tuberculosis, the wrecking of their immune systems by HIV allows the reactivation of their infections which progress rapidly to death – but not before many more tubercle bacilli have been coughed up to contaminate the environment and increase the already great likelihood of an enhanced rate of new infections.

Global warming will almost inevitably lead to increases in tropical diseases, for many of which there are neither preventive vaccines nor therapeutic drugs. Increasing droughts interfering with food production, combined with the excess of population, are likely to precipitate major famines and major outbreaks of epidemic infectious disease carried to regions where they are presently unknown. Such changes would almost certainly set in motion major movements of populations such as have not been seen for almost 2000 years. The press of emigration westwards from Asia and northwards from Africa into Europe, and in the western hemisphere northwards into the USA and Canada, would be difficult, if not impossible, to stem. Among the infections which these migrants would carry with them would certainly be tuberculosis and HIV, itself a prime cause of the increase in tuberculous disease in North America as well as Africa.

Filoviruses – Marburg agent and Ebola virus – which cause highly fatal haemorrhagic diseases, appear unpredictably in Africa, killing many and spreading panic widely. Most outbreaks have been hospital related; transmission seems to be via contact with blood and body fluids of patients. A wildlife reservoir is assumed to exist, but until the ecology of these agents is understood very little can be done to prevent the sporadic epidemic outbreaks which they cause, nor to prevent their spread to the countries of the developed world. Among the large number of people travelling rapidly by air to destinations all over the world, a single person incubating an infection would be able to introduce a highly virulent agent, and begin transmitting it, without any warning being possible. Should a mutation arise capable of infecting by the aerial route the outlook would be exceedingly grave. Rubella virus is a member of the family Togaviridae, which contains many epidemiologically important arthropod-borne viruses such as dengue, yellow fever, and numerous encephalitis viruses. Rubella virus is not vector borne; infection, which requires close person-to-person contact, is probably spread by the aerial route. The possibility of a mutation in a pathogen from one mode of spread to another is always present, and if one should occur in a filovirus, in our present state of knowledge the result could well be catastrophic rather than merely disastrous. Large changes in continental ecology driven by global warming, not only in Africa, but also in Asia and South America, could be responsible for very great alterations in the public health of countries of the developed world.

# Index